Look up other books by:
Dr. Verna R. Benjamin-Lambert

The Healthy Benji book series
Kindergarten through Fifth Grade
On Becoming Your Authentic Self

HEALTH INTELLIGENCE

The Path to a Healthier You

by

Dr. Verna R. Benjamin-Lambert

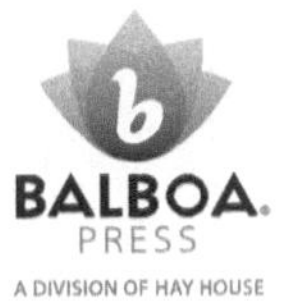

Balboa Press books may be ordered through booksellers or by contacting:

Balboa Press
A Division of Hay House
1663 Liberty Drive
Bloomington, IN 47403
www.balboapress.com
1-(877) 407-4847

Printed in the United States of America.

ISBN: 978-1-4525-7564-3 (sc)
ISBN: 978-1-4525-7566-7 (hc)
ISBN: 978-1-4525-7565-0 (e)
Library of Congress Control Number: 2013910575
Balboa Press rev. date: 03/04/2014

Dedication

The inspiration to write this book came from the courage demonstrated by my daughter Nadia and her husband Ken during the early years of their son Benjamin's life.

When Benjamin was born we celebrated the eagerly anticipated arrival of the family's first grandson. Benjamin was welcomed into a delivery room populated with all three of his aunts, his godmother, and myself—his "Nana." Despite Nadia's very difficult pregnancy, Benjamin arrived on time and with a clean bill of health.

Unfortunately, the exceedingly strong start to life evidenced at the time of Benjamin's birth and in the months that followed would all but disappear by the time Benjamin reached eighteen months old, when he was diagnosed with Pervasive Developmental Disorder. This disorder is most strongly associated with autism.

Because up until the age of ten months Benjamin had met and exceeded his developmental milestones, no one could have imagined a diagnosis of this nature. Benjamin had showed signs of advanced development in the acquisition of language as early as ten months. He would exclaim "good!" whenever he ate food that he thoroughly enjoyed.

Benjamin's behavior started to change dramatically when he turned eleven months old and received a combination of DTP,

DTaP, DT, HIB, and influenza immunizations. Within one week of receiving these immunizations he started to become increasingly detached and disconnected. It was also evident that his cognitive development had become impaired.

Benjamin's mental and emotional decline became a concern to the family. Nadia and Ken took him to the doctor repeatedly to voice their concerns about the changes they were observing, but were consistently told that Benjamin was doing well and that their concerns were unwarranted.

As the months passed, Benjamin's condition greatly deteriorated. He began to experience mild seizures. At night he would cry, kick, and scream endlessly. As the frequency and duration of Benjamin's fits increased, I feared that Nadia and Ken were engaged in a battle that they were not equipped to fight.

At a time when any couple could have succumbed to the confusion, frustration, and utter exhaustion that marked this troubling time in Benjamin's development, Nadia and Ken refused to sit by and be crippled by despair and helplessness, but rather began conducting research to educate themselves about the causes, effects, and possible cures for autism and its related conditions. Soon after they acquired the information about Benjamin's condition they embarked on a mission to employ best practices medically, emotionally, and spiritually to ensure that their son would get better.

At age three Benjamin was showing remarkable progress. By paying close attention to Benjamin's diet and following the instructions of a remarkable and determined naturopathic doctor, his speech and other cognitive functions took on a rapid growth. It's a pleasure to report that at age seven Benjamin is now on grade level academically. He is a well-adjusted child who has brought much joy to our family.

My hope is that Benjamin's story will serve to encourage parents and caregivers not to give up even when the diagnosis seems dismal. I believe that the simple principles outlined in *Health Intelligence* will help to inspire a more health conscious generation of children, families, and health educators.

It's my honor to dedicate this book to Nadia, Ken, and Benjamin.

Acknowledgments

It's with a great sense of pride and gratitude that I thank my mom and dad for their ongoing support throughout the years. Thanks to my husband, Harry, who has consistently stood by my side with his ego in check as he encourages me to follow my dreams wherever they lead. Thanks to my four children—Melissa, Nicole, Nadia and Lauren—who individually and collectively have been my cheerleaders as I expressed my desire to write this book.

Very special thanks to my editors, Dr. Albert A. Benjamin and Thomas Hauck, and my daughter Nicole Kelly for her expertise in refining the manuscript.

Thanks also to Dr. Joanna Robinson for her dedication in helping to bring this book to fruition.

We extend our collective gratitude to First Lady Michelle Obama for drawing attention to the problem of obesity, which is facing an increasing number of families and young people in the United States today.

Table of Contents

INTRODUCTION

"We can all agree that in the wealthiest nation on Earth, all children should have the basic nutrition they need to learn and grow and to pursue their dreams, because in the end, nothing is more important than the health and well-being of our children.... These are the basic values that we all share, regardless of race, party, religion. This is what we share."

— First Lady Michelle Obama at the signing of the Healthy, Hunger-Free Kids Act.

When is a blessing also a curse?

A blessing is having that which you need for your daily sustenance. A curse results when this same blessing is taken to excess so that it becomes toxic. In the United States today, and indeed in many areas of the industrialized world, what was once scarce is now plentiful. Across this great nation where not so long ago starvation was a real threat to life there are now rows of supermarkets and fast-food restaurants, all full to overflowing with nearly every variety of food imaginable. On every corner of every city and suburb, at every highway rest stop, in every mall, Americans can find more food than they could possibly consume, and at bargain prices.

Unfortunately, the food is not always what your grandmother would recognize. Most of it is processed, salted, corn-syruped, freeze-dried, and modified beyond recognition. It's designed to be fast, easy, and cheap. The goal is to fill you up and then make sure you come back for more.

The results of the food explosion have been spectacular—in a very unhealthy way.

In America today, millions of intelligent and well-meaning people—parents, children, rich and poor alike—are becoming obese. Not just well fed, but sick.

Obesity contributes to serious health problems including heart conditions, strokes, cancers, and respiratory problems. Each year, ever-younger children are facing the effects of obesity at rates similar to those found in adults. Obesity is troublesome not only because it affects physical health but also because of its effects on mental health and relationships.

What contributes to the problem of obesity? Individual differences in lifestyle and genetics play a significant role in physical health. Environmental factors also contribute to the obesity epidemic. These factors include the media, advertising, fast food restaurants, the family, parenting, poverty, institutions such as schools, and political agendas.

The present trend of dietary unhealthiness is hurting families. To get back to a healthy lifestyle requires commitment, discipline, and a concerted effort to move towards better health. This shift has to happen not only to improve the health of adults but for the sake of our children and generations to come.

If good health is the goal, healthy eating is only part of the solution. A comprehensive approach to good health requires (a) meaningful relationships, (b) spiritual awareness and practices, (c) environmental wholeness, (d) physical health including nutrition, sleep, dental care, and exercise, and (e) ongoing mental stimulation.

Taken together, this is Health Intelligence.

If we look at the habits of those who have lived to be centurions, we will find that the recipe for longer life consists of a balance. In a recent survey of centurions conducted by United Health Care, the findings showed that 89% communicate with a family member or friend daily. Sixty-seven percent pray or engage in some form of spiritual activity. Fifty-one percent have an exercise regimen that allows them to participate in an activity almost every day. Seventy-one percent sleep for at least eight hours—in contrast to baby boomers, some of whom sleep half that much.

Another significant characteristic of centurions is in their daily eating habits. Over 80% of centurions eat balanced meals, compared to 68% of baby boomers.

We can all learn to improve our lifestyles; we must simply commit to the process and focus on little successes along the way towards better health.

Because social and environmental factors can impact our physical and mental health in dramatic ways, we each need to develop our own Health Intelligence to take control of our health. We need to look at how we learn from these outside resources, how our learning styles affect our choices, how we apply or choose not to apply our knowledge in the real world, and what it ultimately means to be health intelligent. Because knowledge is all around us and we learn from what we see, hear, taste, touch, and feel, it's critical that we explore how we can become more health intelligent.

How can having Health Intelligence make a difference? Intelligence begins with the ability to gather information. With information, individuals can make better choices in everyday life regarding their health. Individuals can analyze, apply, integrate, and draw conclusions about information that can improve their overall lifestyles and mortality outcomes. With a few significant changes, individuals can achieve strong mental health, enjoy greater longevity, have more energy, and experience many other positive outcomes.

In this book, I'll show you how you can develop your Health Intelligence, make better choices, and get more pleasure out of life. It's not hard, and it's something that everyone in the family can understand and make a part of their daily lives. I truly believe that with a well developed sense of Health Intelligence, you'll have more energy, a higher quality of life, and better health for many years to come.

Ready? Let's get started!

Dr. Benji

Chapter 1

Human Intelligence

The measure of intelligence is the ability to change.
— Albert Einstein

Researchers say learning and intelligence are two distinct concepts that work closely together. Learning is the *process* of acquiring new information. Intelligence is the ability to learn, to retain what is learned, and to use logical reasoning to solve problems effectively.

Learning and intelligence in childhood and early adulthood are important predictors of success in obtaining social mobility, adult social status, and income. They are crucial because what we learn and how we use that information are pivotal in understanding human behavior. It's one thing to learn all kinds of information and to have various levels of understanding, but if we don't ever use that knowledge, then what's the point?

Intelligence has been defined in multiple ways. Researchers and theorists have different beliefs about what constitutes intelligence and how it affects everyday life, but there are some generally accepted notions of intelligence that they share. For the purposes of this book, we'll focus on a specific notion of intelligence to see how it can affect our choices, eating habits, overall health, and lifestyles.

Single Intelligence

Two ideas are prominent in the study of intelligence: the notion of a single intelligence factor and the idea that humans have multiple intelligences that contribute to an overall intelligence profile.

Traditionally, researchers have believed that individuals have an overall general intelligence, which is the ability that allows people to process information of any type and in any context. Over time, this approach has grown to dominate psychometric tests (tests that measure intelligence), and it has become widely used and understood as the general factor that describes human mental abilities. Psychometric intelligence (intelligence measured by tests such as the Weschler Intelligence Test and the Stanford-Binet IQ Test) is described as generic thinking skills that include efficient learning, reasoning, problem solving, and abstract thinking.

Researchers have used the idea of a single intelligence to study the relationship between various social factors including education level, achievement, socioeconomic level, health and longevity, and mortality rates. For example, a child's IQ predicts his or her later socioeconomic success more accurately than a parent's attributes. Researchers consistently report that factors such as problem-solving ability, mental speed, general knowledge, creativity, abstract thinking, and memory all play key roles in the measure and standard of intelligence, suggesting that a quality of intelligence is the ability to interact with the environment and overcome its challenges.

Multiple Intelligences

General intelligence is only one way of looking at intelligence. Humans have a variety of mental capacities, and not all are captured by the concept of a single intelligence. Over time, we have come to accept multiple definitions of intelligence, suggesting that abilities other than the traditionally studied mathematics and linguistic abilities are valuable in society. We value individuals who possess unique abilities in sports, music, interpersonal relationships, intrapersonal understanding, and a variety of other areas.

In the 1980s, researchers proposed the idea that people learn and think differently and therefore possess *multiple intelligences* rather than one general intelligence. This idea was appealing to educators, who could see that children were displaying a wide range of abilities and strengths in the classroom. Educators realized that there must be an alternate way to explain the differences in learning and acquisition of knowledge. One general intelligence factor was no longer satisfactory in explaining learning; instead, researchers and educators turned to the idea that multiple intelligences could explain the variation in human abilities. This was used to promote a more diverse approach to teaching and learning in which diverse strengths are supported and individuals are encouraged to improve upon their weaknesses.

Harvard University professor Howard Gardner initially identified seven intelligences and later modified his list to include an eighth. The following chart helps define the intelligences in detail by indicating the behavioral strengths, preferred activities, and learning style associated with each type of intelligence. Although all humans possess all of the intelligences to some degree, individuals can show more strength in one or more intelligence areas.

Intelligence Area:	Is Strong In:	Likes to:	Learns Best Through:	Famous Examples:
1. Verbal-Linguistic (Word Smart)	reading, writing, telling stories, memorizing dates, thinking words	read, write, tell stories, talk, memorize, work at puzzles	reading, hearing, and seeing words, speaking, writing, discussing and debating	T.S. Eliot, Maya Angelou, Virginia Woolf, Abraham Lincoln
2. Math-Logic (Number Smart)	math, reasoning, logic, problem-solving, patterns	solve problems, question, work with numbers, experiment	working with patterns and relationships, classifying, categorizing, working with the abstract	Albert Einstein, John Dewey, Susanne Langer
3. Spatial (Picture Smart)	reading, maps, charts, drawing, mazes, puzzles, making images, visualization	design, draw, build, create, daydream, look at pictures	working with pictures and colors, visualizing, using the mind's eye, drawing	Pablo Picasso, Frank Lloyd Wright, Georgia O'Keeffe, Bobby Fischer
4. Bodily-Kinesthetic (Body Smart)	athletics, dancing, acting, crafts, using tools	move around, touch and talk, use body language	touching, moving, processing knowledge through bodily sensations	Charlie Chaplin, Martina Navratilova, Magic Johnson

5. Musical (Music Smart)	singing, picking up sounds, remembering melodies, rhythms	sing, hum, play an instrument, listen to music	rhythm, melody, singing, listening to music and melodies	Leonard Bernstein, Wolfgang Amadeus Mozart, Ella Fitzgerald
6. Interpersonal (People Smart)	understanding people, leading, organizing, communicating, resolving conflicts, selling	have friends, talk to people, join groups	sharing, comparing, relating, interviewing, cooperating	Mohandas Gandhi, Ronald Reagan, Mother Theresa
7. Intrapersonal (Self Smart)	understanding self, recognizing strengths and weaknesses, setting goals	work alone, reflect, pursue interests	working alone, doing self-paced projects, having space, reflecting	Eleanor Roosevelt, Sigmund Freud, Thomas Merton
8. Naturalist (Nature Smart)	understanding nature, making distinctions, identifying flora and fauna	be involved with nature, make distinctions	working in nature, exploring living things, learning about plants and natural events	John Muir, Charles Darwin, Luther Burbank

Whether you believe in the idea of one general intelligence or prefer to conceptualize human abilities as multiple intelligences, intelligence is a factor that affects your daily choices, your eating habits, your approach to tasks, your relationships with others, your understanding and ability to process new information, your preference for activities, and ultimately, your future.

Some educators and researchers believe intelligence can be understood from only one of the two approaches—the general intelligence approach or the multiple intelligence approach. However, it's not necessary to focus on one approach to the exclusion of the other. Both approaches can offer significant insight and direction in understanding the concept of a new intelligence—Health Intelligence.

What Is Health Intelligence?

At the core of problematic health trends such as the obesity epidemic lies a lack of basic understanding of what it means to be healthy. Some individuals who have healthy eating and exercise habits have difficulty understanding why such a high percentage of individuals in our society have become so unhealthy. But being healthy is not just a matter of avoiding that which we know to be unhealthy. Rather, to be healthy we need to use what I call *Health Intelligence*—a ninth category to be added to the intelligence spectrum.

Health Intelligence is understanding, developing and implementing healthy routines to produce a wholesome and productive lifestyle.

Health Intelligence integrates knowledge about the body, soul, and mind. To be health intelligent, all areas of the individual's being must be addressed equally, cared for equally, and nurtured equally. No one area is more valuable than another, and all three areas are necessary for positive overall health. Without a balance between the three areas, overall health is at risk. A visual representation of Health Intelligence would look something like the following diagram:

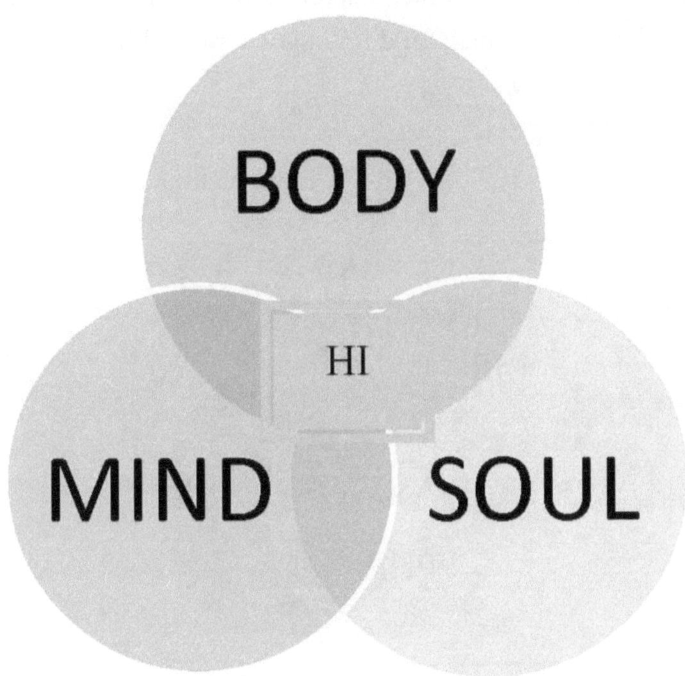

Howard Gardner (1999) the originator of the theory of multiple intelligences, believed the purpose of schooling "should be to develop intelligences and to help people reach vocational and avocational goals that are appropriate to their particular spectrum of intelligences" (p.34). People who are empowered in this way feel more engaged and competent and are therefore more inclined to serve society in a constructive way. I certainly support this belief.

I further believe that having the ability to live a healthy life is *not an inborn trait*. Healthy living is an *acquired behavior* that must be taught and developed effectively through education, modeling, practice, and discipline.

As previously stated, healthy eating is not enough to guarantee total health. We must also have: (a) meaningful relationships, (b) spiritual awareness and practices, (c) environmental wholeness, (d) physical health regimens, and (e) ongoing mental stimulation. See the diagram below.

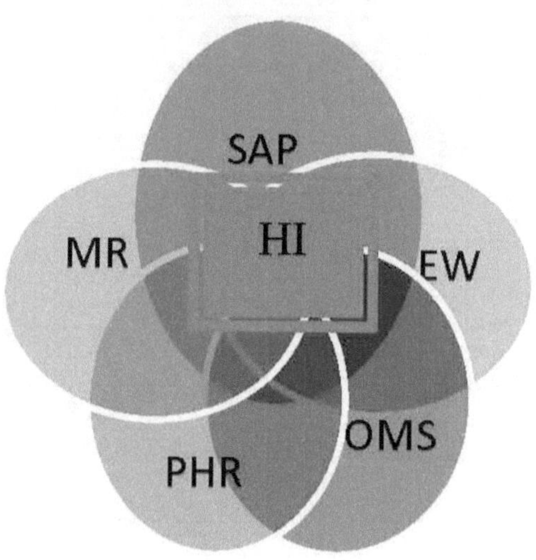

Total health means that all of these areas are addressed appropriately in the individual's life so he or she is living a well-rounded, well-balanced existence. If one area is neglected, the whole individual suffers, and health becomes a concern. Overall good health requires a happy balance of these five lifestyle areas.

There is an abundance of research on the different effects of physical illness, disease, doctor care, nutrition, and daily lifestyle. People are becoming more and more willing to take steps to improve their physical health. In addition, people often choose to address physical pain, illness, and disease before other facets of the important balance (for example, soul and mind) simply because they are concrete problems that can often be readily addressed.

The job of the patient is becoming more complex, and individuals have to deal with new, ever-changing, and multifaceted information on what is required to care for their own health and the health of their families. Researchers have confirmed that inadequate thinking skills can get in the way of effective self-care. To keep up with complicated and rapidly evolving health information, we need to use critical-thinking skills. Unfortunately, a large segment of society has not been taught how to use these more advanced thinking skills.

People go to the doctor all the time for basic care and routine checkups. Doctors prescribe specific medicines or other care that is meant to promote healthiness and well-being. Doctors have the best interests of the patient in mind and want to give that patient necessary information and strategies for self-care. But what are the chances that people actually follow through on the recommendations at home? Maybe they do, and maybe they do not.

The important question is: Why don't people always follow their doctor's orders?

Many patients ignore their doctors' orders not because of their unwillingness to comply, but because they lack the training to do so. These patients may not understand the directions and may not be able to implement the recommended treatments, especially as regimens become more complex. There is simply too much to remember: which prescriptions to take, what time to take each of them, whether to take them with or without food, what dietary restrictions each requires, and so forth. All of these extra details add to the complexity of the recommendations and leave patients feeling overwhelmed, increasing the risk of noncompliance. This is especially true for those who are more advanced in age.

When people can't absorb or remember the information they need, their health suffers.

In this environment, Health Intelligence is more crucial than ever. What does this mean exactly? It means that individuals have to be smart about everyday health choices. That includes being intelligent about alcohol, drug, or cigarette consumption; food choices; eating habits; nutritional information; dental habits; physical activity choices; sleeping habits; mental health care; spiritual health; relationships; spiritual care; and every other aspect of health. That is a lot to consider, but the combination of healthy behaviors is related to understanding health information and being able to apply it to everyday decision making about health. It means taking care of all the different facets of your life so that you are living a wise, balanced, and happy life.

Choosing Knowledge

Because the media regularly reports new health information everyone has a chance to obtain it, but equal *access* to information does not necessarily mean equal *understanding*. Surprisingly, when more knowledge about health risks and new diagnostic options are made public, the people who seem to be most responsive to the new information are those who are already relatively well-informed about health issues. By the same token, a person who is more Health Intelligent will not necessarily be more compliant with treatment or exhibit healthier behavior. Research evidence shows that a person's Health Intelligence can be linked to hospitalization, the number and severity of current illnesses, annual medical costs, and self-rated health.

Overall, people with higher health training tend to report better health. If people with higher test scores are more likely than those with a lower educational level to undergo routine medical checkups and screenings, they are also more likely to have health problems discovered and diagnosed. This means that problems can be treated sooner and, potentially, the treatments can be more effective. Additionally, prevention measures can be applied when familial patterns of health problems are discovered early. Being Health Intelligent can benefit the patient, the immediate family, the extended family, and even the larger society, which benefits from necessary, timely, and affordable health care for its members.

Regardless of your current knowledge about health issues and your educational level, you can still learn more. It's not too late to become informed and interested in your own health. Anyone can learn. If you are open to improving your self-care, if you want to be in better health, and if you are interested in improved wellbeing for you and your family, you can learn. If you are ready to begin the journey into improved Health Intelligence, read on.

THE BODY

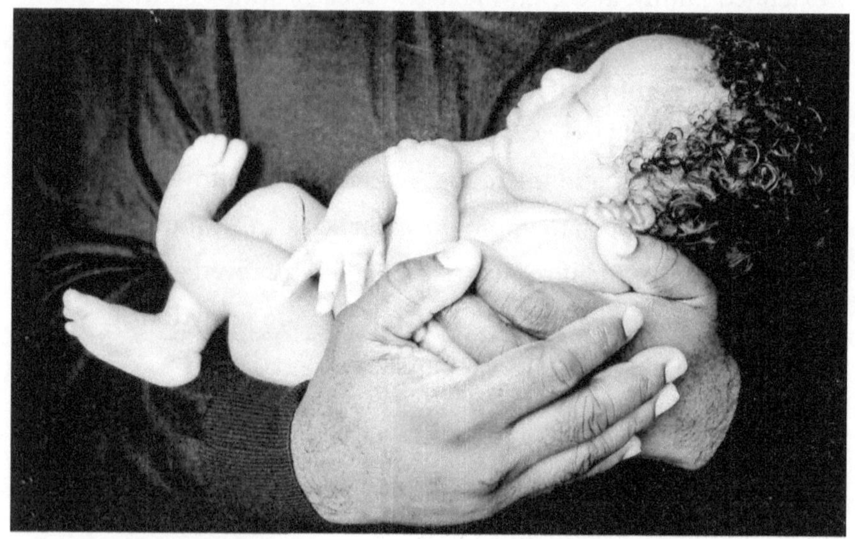

Courtesy of Libbie Wicket

There are two ways to live your life. One is
as though nothing is a miracle. The other
is as though everything is a miracle.

— Albert Einstein

Chapter 2

The Body

It is confidence in our bodies, minds and spirits that allows us to keep looking for new adventures, new directions to grow in, and new lessons to learn - which is what life is all about.
— Oprah Winfrey

The human body is the most extraordinary creation. Even more astonishing is that it's made up of approximately 70% of water and four key elements—hydrogen, oxygen, carbon, and nitrogen. In order for it to function effectively, along with these elements the body must be nourished with food that is rich in vitamins, iron, protein, carbohydrates, and fat. If all of these elements are not present to support the balanced sustenance of life, over time, serious malfunction occurs. If medical intervention or a change in the way the body is treated is not taken to correct such imbalances, numerous types of illnesses can result that could possibly lead to death.

Obviously, each of us needs to take care of our body. We need to understand what it needs to function so that good health can be maintained and achieved. In the process of understanding our body, we each need a clear lens that allows us to look and reflect on it both from the inside and outside.

The first step in achieving the goal of body care is to make a conscious choice to take ownership of your body, because you alone are responsible for taking care of this great structure. Once ownership is acknowledged, its care should include nutrition, exercise, dental health, compliance with medical care, and protection from over exposure from the sun. In addition, we need to make daily lifestyle choices that will sustain general body functions.

Nutrition

The body needs nutrients for the sustenance of life. We are well aware that there are countless numbers of foods in the marketplace that have no nutritional value. We cannot become complacent; we must make every effort to find the foods that will provide the nourishment that the body needs to keep us healthy. A lifetime of nutritious eating means focusing on consuming healthy foods every day that will prevent deficiencies of vitamins, iron, and other minerals. It means eating foods that are low in carbohydrates and fat. It means eating foods that will aid in supplying the brain with nutrients that will provide us with clarity of thought. It means enjoying healthy beverages. It means making sure that when we indulge ourselves, we do so only in moderation.

In today's consumer-oriented economy where we have large quantities of food available wherever and whenever we want, maintaining a proper diet requires discipline. This can be hard to maintain if both reward and consequence are not foremost in our mind. Some of us consistently complain that there is not enough time or energy left after working eight hours to prepare a balanced meal at home; therefore, eating out becomes the norm. Similar reasons are given for the lack of exercise and inadequate sleep. These excuses are causing illness and disease at alarming rates, not only in this country but internationally.

Exercise

The relationship of exercise to the body is as crucial as breathing is to life. Exercise provides much needed support for the muscles, glands, cells, skeletal framework, and organs, and helps the respiratory system to function healthily. The body depends on exercise to strengthen the heart and bones, and for the rejuvenation of cells. The increase of oxygenated blood that is enhanced by exercise serves to nourish, promote growth, and enrich the mind. Without an exercise regimen the body experiences a slow decline that will ultimately cause shortening of the lifespan.

Whenever we hear about healthy eating, we also hear about the importance of exercise. It's true that the two concepts go hand in hand to achieve the most effective and comprehensive results. Just like healthy eating, exercising every day is a lifestyle choice that requires commitment, focus, and motivation. It's necessary to keep our calories in check even as we exercise. Most research suggests that adults should exercise at least thirty minutes per day, whereas children should exercise about sixty minutes each day. Some basic exercise ideas that can help you make smart choices about what to do and what not to do are:

1. Exercise should be fun, age-specific, and tailored to the individual's fitness level and ability.
2. Exercise should involve large muscle groups to increase energy expenditure.

3. Exercise should increase in frequency, intensity, and duration with time.
4. You should restrict sedentary behaviors (for example, television viewing, video games, and Internet surfing).

When beginning any exercise regimen, it's important to start slowly and build up to a higher level of intensity as you go. It's critical not to overwork the muscles so that you get sore and lose the desire to continue. Start with walking and then gradually advance to more intense cardiovascular activities. Turn walking into a slight jog or try a walking and sprinting combination workout. Also, focus on a variety of movements. Try sit-ups and push-ups, or play tennis, soccer, basketball, or other sports that impact different muscle groups. Change it up to keep exercise entertaining and well-rounded for the body.

As an exercise regime is established, it's a good idea to follow these guidelines. Because a pre-workout snack is advantageous for fueling, eat before exercising. Choose carbohydrates and protein so that you'll burn more calories. It goes without saying, but always be sure to fuel and refuel with water after a workout. Staying hydrated is critical to overall health because of the effects it has on detoxing the body and replenishing the system after the loss of fluid.

If you think you don't have the time or motivation to work out consistently, there are several easy ways that you can incorporate exercise into your everyday routine without much effort. For example, when you park your car, don't circle around your destination until you find the closest parking spot; instead, park farther away and walk a few extra steps to burn a few extra calories. When you're watching television, stand up and walk in place during the commercials, and you may burn as many calories as you would if you took a walk. During one hour, you can take roughly 2,100 steps and burn 150 calories. Do sit-ups, push-ups, leg lifts, or abdominal crunches during the commercials. Don't always take the elevator; take the stairs sometimes. Don't set items on the stairs to take up later; take them up immediately and get in the extra steps.

These are just a few simple ways to build in extra steps to expend more energy, which can make a substantial difference to your overall health.

Sleep and Rest

Sleep is a state of unconsciousness during which the mind and body slow down and are rejuvenated. It's a true escape from worry, anxiety, pain, and the responsibilities of life that haunt us during waking hours. Even the most controlling individual cannot escape this process unless the gift of sleep is taken from him. In the words of Miguel de Cervantes, "Now, blessings light on him that first invented sleep! It covers a man all over, thoughts and all like a cloak; it's meat for the hungry, drink for the thirsty, heat for the cold, and cold for the hot. It's the current coin that purchases all the pleasures of the world cheap, and the balance that sets the king and the shepherd, the fool and the wise man, even."

Good sleep slows down the aging process and contributes to overall happiness. Lack of sleep will result in the deterioration of the mind, body and nerves. Some individuals do not need as much sleep as others, but everyone needs sleep.

Recommended Sleep by Age

Age	Total Sleep Needed	Additional Notes
1-4 Weeks	15-16 Hours	Newborns are developing their internal biological clocks.
1-4 Months	14-15 Hours	Regular sleeping patterns begin and longer night sleeping.
4-12 Months	14-15 Hours	Important to establish regular sleeping patterns at this time.
1-3 Years	12-14 Hours	Naps remain important to sleep health.
3-6 Years	10-12 Hours	Naps will become shorter.
7-12 Years	10-11 Hours	Bedtime gets later.
12-18 Years	8-9 Hours	Teens may need more sleep.
Adults	7-8 Hours	Times will greatly vary.
Pregnant	8+	More sleep and naps may be needed.

Source: http://www.sleepaidresource.com/sleep-chart.html

Just as our body needs exercise for good health, it also needs rest and proper sleep to rejuvenate us and replenish the energy needed for everyday tasks. People tend to underestimate the value and importance of sleeping eight hours per night, but if you knew the benefits of a decent night's sleep, along with the obvious negative side effects of a poor night's sleep, you might think twice about your sleeping habits. Obviously, poor sleeping habits can lead to excessive daytime sleepiness; although it's uncomfortable to be sleepy during the day, this kind of continued sleepiness can be related to the diminished memory and thinking skills, a condition in older people known as cognitive decline.

Beyond making you cranky, irritable, easily frustrated, and easily annoyed, sleep deprivation can have some other negative effects. People who average no more than six hours of sleep per night may have a higher risk of diabetes and heart disease. These individuals may be more likely to eat more and gain more weight. Additionally, people who have limited sleep or disrupted sleep eat an average of three hundred more calories per day than those who sleep as long as they want.

Poor sleep patterns have also been associated with mental deterioration and Alzheimer's disease. Poor sleep patterns are especially a problem for people with sleep apnea. Essentially, people with sleep apnea stop breathing several times a night and, therefore, have consistently disturbed sleep patterns. These individuals are much more likely to develop mild thinking problems or dementia than problem-free sleepers.

If you have sleeping problems, get them checked out and work on a solution. Some solutions that should be considered common knowledge deserve repeating, including getting regular exercise and avoiding caffeine and alcohol. Exercising regularly can improve sleep. Caffeine and nicotine can dramatically interfere with sleep; caffeine is a stimulant that can affect you up to sixteen hours after you consume it. Alcohol can affect sleep. Although it may be effective in initially inducing sleep, alcohol impairs sleep during the second half of the night, thus reducing overall sleep time. As a result, alcohol use can also cause daytime sleepiness.

There are some basic, free, and sensible ways to get better sleep. Professionals suggest the following:

1. Sticking to a consistent sleep schedule (always going to bed and waking up around the same time, even on weekends and holidays).

2. Relaxing before bed and practicing a calming bedtime ritual that does not include television, video games, or work.
3. Watching what you eat or drink before bed. This includes sugar, caffeine, alcohol, heavy foods, and spicy foods. Some of these substances can interfere with breathing and the ability to fall asleep and stay asleep. Others can cause sleep-disrupting disorders such as restless legs, stomach upset, and acid reflux.
4. Creating a bedroom that is cool, dark, and quiet. Choose a comfortable bed, sheets, pillow, and pajamas.
5. Avoiding daytime naps that can interfere with nighttime sleep.
6. Finding healthy ways to manage stress during the day so you can rest at night.

Dental Care

Good dental hygiene is critical to the overall health of the body. Not only can it provide clues to certain body illnesses such as diabetes, oral cancer, pancreatic cancer, leukemia, and kidney disease, but it can also prevent the onset of diseases such as gingivitis, swollen gums, and low birth weight in babies. It's therefore essential to consider dental care as part of the overall process of taking care of your body. As noted previously, daily dental care can prevent significant problems, and regular visits to the dentist can ensure that your mouth is healthy. It's extremely important to brush your teeth at least twice per day. Daily flossing and a rinse with a good mouthwash should become a part of your daily routine.

Certain dietary changes can also improve the quality of the teeth and mouth. Cutting down on sugar in the form of candy, sweets, and soda beverages can lead to a reduction in cavities. Maintaining a diet that is high in calcium is another smart way to improve the strength and condition of the teeth. While calcium can be found in many foods, those that are high in calcium include dried herbs, cheese, sesame seeds, tofu, almonds, flax seeds, dairy products, green leafy vegetables, herring, and Brazil nuts.

Protecting the Body and Basic Safety

In addressing the needs of the physical body, there are a number of other pertinent considerations. In addition to healthy eating, exercise, and proper sleep, basic safety and the protection of the body are essential. Taking care of our physical body means being aware of our surroundings and protecting all parts of our body from harm. To be health intelligent about protecting the body, you should do the following:

1. Visit your doctor regularly for checkups and preventive care.
2. Follow your doctor's orders. Take prescription medications as directed, and follow your doctor's suggestions about diet, exercise, and sleep.
3. Use sunscreen. Use one ounce, which is a golf ball size or the amount that fits into a shot glass. Using SPF 30, rather than 15, will make a substantial difference in its effectiveness.
4. Get plenty of fresh air, fresh water, and sunshine.
5. Wear your seatbelt and drive defensively.
6. Wear safety goggles, a bike helmet, knee pads, sunglasses, rubber gloves, and other safety equipment as needed.
7. Avoid illegal drugs, cigarettes, deadly weapons, toxic chemicals, and other dangerous materials.

8. Use alcohol moderately and responsibly.
9. Have protected, safe, healthy, and monogamous sex.
10. Learn basic first aid and CPR so you are prepared for any emergency.
11. Address any problems or health concerns when you notice them; do not wait.

Taking care of the physical body is an everyday task. Our bodies include hundreds of working parts that require constant care and attention. We should frequently assess ourselves for health-related changes. If there is a change in what was once normal for us, we should observe it, learn more about it, and seek help from a professional who can provide us with additional information to enhance our Health Intelligence that can lead to a solution.

Taking care of the body is one of the most crucial things you can do to move toward Health Intelligence. The second thing you can do is pay attention to the mind, which is the intellectual and emotional center of our being.

THE BRAIN & MIND CONNECTION

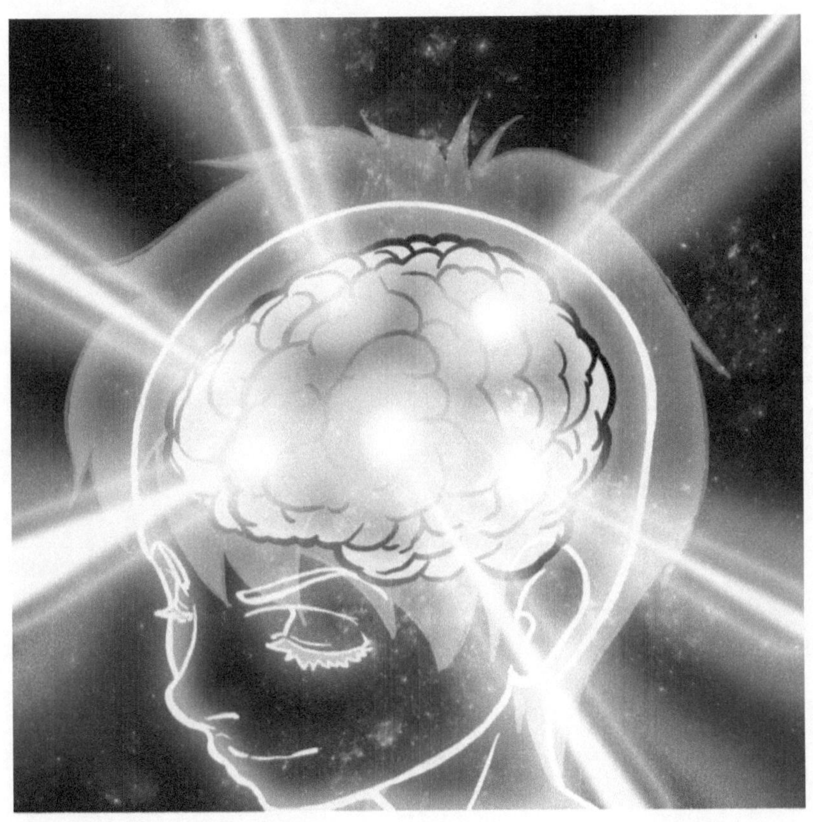

CHAPTER 3

The Mind

The power of the mind is your power. Use it. Don't let it use you.

—Terri Guillemet

The mind functions within the brain. The brain is designed like an extraordinarily complex computer that is wired to support all body functions. It's quite a mysteriously designed piece of hardware that science has yet to duplicate. For this book, I will describe the brain as being the hardware with the mind being the operating system that conveys the messages to be interpreted through the use of the senses (seeing, smelling, tasting, hearing, touching). It's then fair to say that the mind is the governing body for all experiences, whether the experience exists in the conscious or unconscious state. The information that is stored in our mind is learned from environmental exposure, genetic predispositions, nature, academia, and through nurturing. All of these factors ultimately determine our success or failures throughout our lifespan.

Because the brain is the seat of emotion and intellect, in order for the mind to function, the brain (hardware) must be nourished so that those impulses can be generated effectively. If the brain deteriorates, the mind will reflect the same level of deterioration. When the brain dies the mind also dies.

If you are able to manage the physical body effectively, you are more likely to have time to exert effort to improve your emotional and intellectual status. As researcher Abraham Maslow suggested, we must first meet the basic requirements for food, shelter, water, sex, air, and clothing before pursuing needs associated with emotional health. Additionally, before we can reach self-actualization we must feel safe, a sense of love and belonging, and esteem. Maslow defined his categories in a hierarchy that builds on the previous level. He suggested the following pyramid:

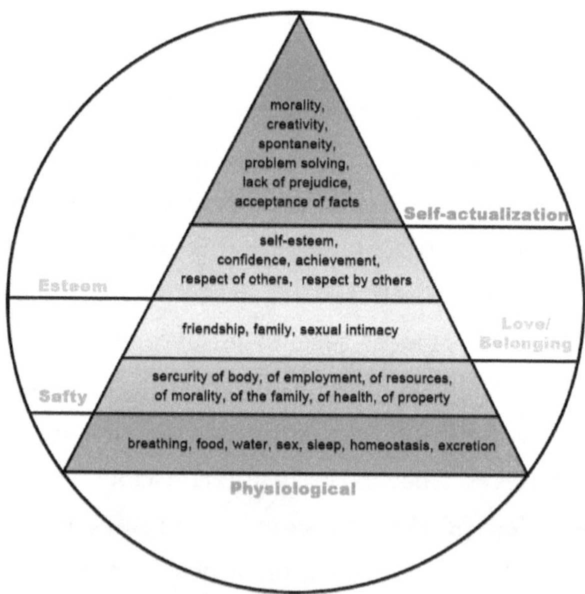

Maslow's Hierarchy of Needs

A homeless or hungry person is consumed by thoughts about finding the next meal, locating clean water, and obtaining a clean place to rest, and is less concerned about morality or self-esteem. When basic needs are met, the individual is more capable of finding safety, security, love, and belonging with others, as well as confidence and respect for himself. We can safely focus on nurturing mental health, improving relationships, and following intellectual pursuits only when the physical body is functioning effectively.

Intellectual Stimulation

Our minds are challenged every day. We must remember facts and data, integrate new material with old information, analyze, synthesize, solve problems, and perform a thousand other intellectual tasks. We process information all the time; we make intellectual connections and we simplify the overwhelming amount of content that is available. We are constantly working to improve how we learn, how we retain information, and how we can make the best use of the information we have. At our best, we continue to pursue intellectual endeavors that enrich our mind and the minds of others. Stimulating the mind in new ways is a necessary facet of Health Intelligence. Without stimulation and change, our actions become repetitive and our minds stagnate. We need to challenge ourselves consistently with content that stimulates the mind.

Although some of us pay attention to our emotions and the health of the mind, I would imagine that there are many people who neglect this area of the self because it is not concrete, tangible, or obvious. Dealing with emotions, coping with stress, and managing relationships can be very intimate; therefore, people are more likely to keep personal experiences to themselves. Some simply choose not to share these personal experiences with anyone, whereas others may believe that it's not important, relevant, or even necessary to do so. In fact, it's essential, relevant, *and* necessary. Taking care of your mental health is part of the overall care of the self; it's one of the five facets of being Health Intelligent.

Making Meaningful Connections

Relationships come and go. You change jobs and coworkers, you move out of the old neighborhood where your neighbors were your friends, you modify your extracurricular activities to include a new crowd. Perhaps you no longer hang out with your friends from high school or college and you've met new friends (as a mom or dad) through your play date crew. Whatever the case, relationships change throughout a person's lifetime. You grow away from some people and closer to others. If you are lucky, you have a few genuine close, personal friends on whom you can truly depend. They might even be your siblings, your parents, or other close relatives.

Strong relationships are necessary for positive mental health. These are the people you trust and enjoy spending time with. These are also the people with whom you have made meaningful connections and with whom you engage in mutual sharing about the self. Undoubtedly, they will be there for you when you need them. Strong relationships are about more than just someone to chat with on the phone, text, or go to a bar or shop with. Everyone needs at least one relationship that has a deep, intimate, and personal connection with an honest and open exchange of feelings and experiences.

Whether it's a friend, a spouse, a mother, a cousin, or a neighbor, maintaining a relationship with someone is hard work. You must invest time, emotion, sometimes money, and a whole lot of yourself in the process. If the relationship is important to both of you, it will not seem like work; it will seem like a step toward something for the greater good of both parties. Taking the time to share your life with someone you care about and who cares about you in return allows for validation of your experiences, feelings, and your whole self. Validation by another person fosters the feelings of safety, security, and self-confidence that are necessary for mental health. Without that kind of support, a person can become unhappy, dissatisfied, lonely, depressed, and ashamed of himself or herself. Validation from a significant other is critical.

Self-Actualization

While validation from others is important, it's equally necessary that we learn how to be our own best friend. Once we feel secure with those around us and are strong enough to learn about the self, we can begin to nurture it. Just like any other relationship, taking care of the self and of our emotions requires commitment, an investment of time, and focus. To take care of the self, we must learn about our feelings, our strengths and weaknesses, what is important to us, and what we need emotionally to survive. The human journey toward personal growth and self-actualization is one that requires ongoing internal nurturing and support.

There are many ways we can work toward self-actualization. We can read self-help books, work with a personal life coach to set work or personal goals, invest in various personal growth activities such as retreats and seminars, share our experiences with a counselor, attend church services, or choose to take any other cooperative journey toward self-awareness and understanding. These guided methods can be immensely helpful and supportive in the process of self-discovery.

Other people might choose an introverted, reflective path

that includes an intimate, personal exploration of emotions and experiences. This may involve activities such as journaling or creative writing, art and art therapy, meditation, yoga, or prayer. These activities can inspire, motivate, and nurture the self.

Regardless of the chosen method, spending time alone, focusing on the self, learning about emotions, and finding new ways to approach self-actualization are necessary for personal growth. This kind of intense self-care is an essential part of Health Intelligence.

Regardless of the path you choose, building a better, healthier you is all about taking care of the body, soul, and mind. These three facets of growth include improved relationships, validation from others, increased self-awareness, support of the self, reflection on emotions and experiences, and a positive swing toward self-actualization. As Abraham Maslow pointed out, it's essential to have our needs for physiological, safety, belonging, esteem, and self-actualization met so that we can to experience fulfillment. We must not disregard the needs of the body, mind, or soul because they must all work synergistically to achieve a wholesome and healthy life.

Feed Your Brain

How you fuel your brain makes a difference in its performance. Everyone knows the old saying, "You are what you eat." If you eat only wholesome foods, it will be reflected in how your body ages over time. Here's a recommended list of foods that supply the brain with the necessary nutrients:

1. Blueberries—Blueberries serve a wide range of functions for improving mental performance. Most notably, regular blueberry consumption has been shown to improve memory function.

Furthermore, blueberries are rich in antioxidants, helping to prevent free radical damage. Still not convinced? Research has found that blueberries can also reverse age related declines in motor function, balance, and coordination.

2. Salmon—Rich in Omega-3 fatty acids, salmon helps your brain develop tissue for increasing your brain power. Furthermore, salmon also plays a key role in fighting Alzheimer's and other age-related cognitive disorders.

3. Flax seeds—Flax seeds are crammed with ALA, a healthy fat that helps the cerebral cortex function more effectively. This is the portion of the brain responsible for processing sensory information. Keeping it sharp is vital.

4. Coffee—Regular coffee drinking has been shown to reduce the risk of Alzheimer's, dementia, and other mental disorders. That's because when used in moderation caffeine is good for the brain, and it contains antioxidants. The important thing to note is you shouldn't add extra ingredients to your coffee, such as those caramel enhancements that are crammed with sweeteners and fatty products.

5. Mixed nuts—Peanuts, walnuts, pecans, and other nuts contain properties that help with everything from fighting insomnia to promoting mental clarity and strong memory. Walnuts are rich in Omega-3 fatty acids, while almonds contain natural mood-enhancing neurotransmitters.

6. Avocados—Don't let the avocado's fat content fool you. It's a healthy fat that promotes blood flow, which keeps your mind functioning at its peak. That's not all—avocados have also been shown to reduce blood pressure.

7. Eggs—Egg yolks are rich in choline, an essential nutrient to improve memory function.

8. Whole grains—From oatmeal to whole grain bread, whole grains are excellent brain foods as they improve circulation and contain essential fiber, vitamins, and even some Omega-3. Don't just choose bread that's labeled *whole wheat*; be sure to make your sandwiches from *whole grain* breads to enjoy the benefits.

9. Chocolate—For me, this is the yummiest brain food of all. Dark chocolate is antioxidant-rich and improves focus and concentration. Milk chocolate, on the other hand, improves memory and reaction time.

10. Broccoli—Broccoli has been shown to improve memory function as well as slow the aging process. This means a broccoli-rich diet will help keep you young and sharp.

THE DNA AND SOUL CONNECTION

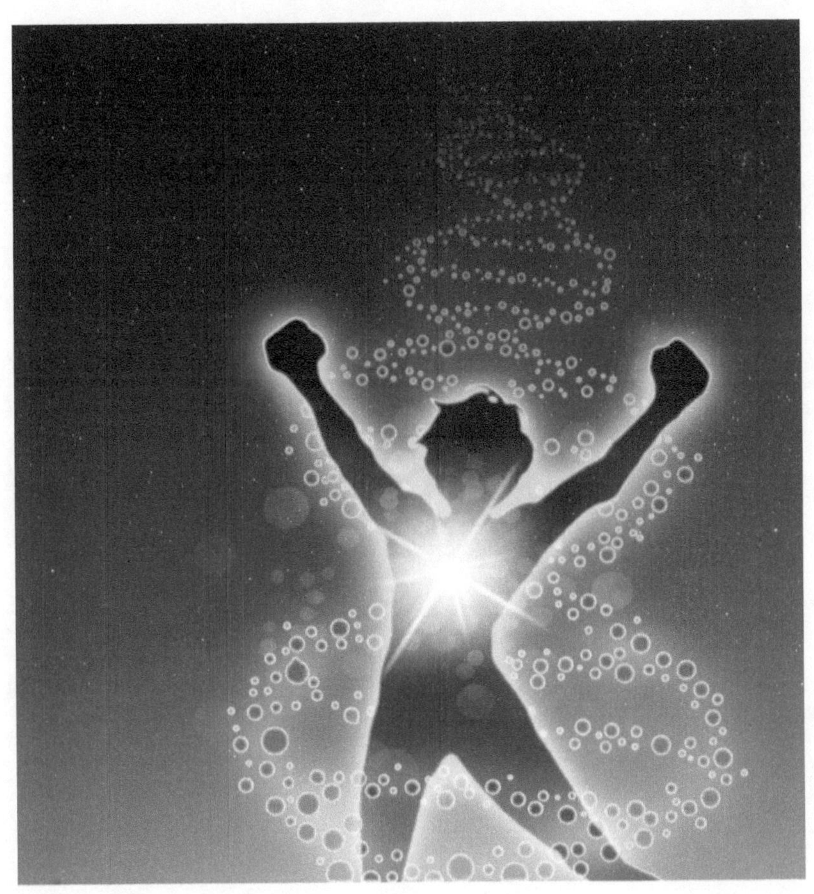

Chapter 4

The Soul and Spirituality

THE SOUL

The Soul, the Electrifying Sparkle of God Within Us
Fills the Body with Eternal Light
Sourced From God the Father
Planted at the Core of Our Being
Sustaining the Body as God Sustains the World
Burning Undimmable Flame
Pure as God. Eternal as God.
Invisible Tree Flourishing With Fruit of Thought
Yielding Gratefulness and Praise
Pruned With Prayer and Meditation It Thrives
Shines through the Heart
Like Bright Light on Pure Diamond
Human Kind Cannot Contain It Because
It Contains Human Kind
Guiding Our Minds and Spirits
Filling the Body Until the Flesh Fails
Returning unto God the Creator
— Dr. Verna R. Benjamin-Lambert

The soul is that spiritual DNA that connects each of us to God. It's unique to each person, but it's also the common denominator that all human beings share. In the same way that our DNA connects us to families in a unique way, the soul connects us to God.

It's fair to say that we all have a piece of God within us.

The soul is a unique presence that governs emotions and rational thought. The body is subject to death, but the soul is not. Just as God is eternal, so too is the soul because it is a part of God. It never dies.

According to the twelfth-century German philosopher Hildegard of Bingen, "The soul is the greening life force of the flesh, for the body grows and prospers through her, just as the earth becomes fruitful when it is moistened. The soul humidifies the body so that it does not dry out, just like the rain which soaks into the earth."

In order for the soul to be fed, there must be time for meditation, prayer, or reflection on giving thanks for all things that are good and lovely. It's a time to search for inner peace and rebuilding of inner strength. Some may engage in such a practice multiple times daily, whereas others may choose once daily. Whatever the frequency may be, the soul must be fed regularly for ultimate achievement of a wholesome life.

Spirituality

Unlike the soul, spirituality is a state of being that can be developed to make meaningful connections to God. The soul is fed and enriched through ones spiritual practices. Frequent engagement in prayer, worship and meditation, provides the path for self-discovery.

Through spirituality, love for self and others, inner peace, joy, tolerance, a spirit of forgiveness, consistent expression of gratitude, kindness, empathy and other acts of kindness are manifested. All the aforementioned attributes must be present in order for anyone to experience a wholesome and healthy life. The lack of spiritual awareness leads to despondency, hopelessness, misery, and a feeling of helplessness.

Suggestions for developing spiritual health include:

✓ Meditate at least fifteen minutes daily.
✓ Maintain a daily gratitude journal.
✓ Perform at least one act of kindness daily.
✓ Begin and end the day by giving thanks to God for His goodness.
✓ Give thanks for each meal.
✓ Share positive experiences with family and friends.
✓ Do not dwell on the negative.
✓ Read a scripture verse daily.
✓ Always lend a helping hand to someone in need (this could be words of encouragement, a ride to work/grocery store/doctor's office). It does not have to be money. Let it be something that you are comfortable doing.
✓ Be polite to individuals you meet or with whom you interact.
✓ Worship with others if it suits your lifestyle.
✓ Pray for the sick, aged, children, homeless, and hungry.
✓ Always tell your significant other "I love you" before you leave home.
✓ Keep a song of praise in your heart.
✓ Above all apply LEN to your daily life:

LOVE YOURSELF

ENRICH YOUR MIND

NOURISH YOUR SOUL.

CHAPTER 5

The Obesity Crisis

Excess generally causes reaction, and produces a change in the opposite direction, whether it be in the seasons, or in individuals, or in governments.
— Plato

In recent times we have seen a frightening increase in adolescent and childhood diseases including obesity, cancer, learning disorders, diabetes, and heart disease.

A significant cause of these afflictions is unhealthy eating.

Most disturbing of these health hazards is the obesity crisis. Since 1980, the obesity rates in the United States have tripled. Americans have long been identified as consumers who indulge and overindulge in fast food and processed food, and who upgrade their servings to oversized portions. With an obesity rate of 30% the United States has a critical problem; however, the obesity epidemic is no longer exclusively an American problem. Individuals in other countries are now affected at similar rates as the United States. According to the Organization for Economic Co-operation and Development (OECD), the countries with the highest obesity rates are the United States, Mexico, the United Kingdom, Slovakia,

Greece, Australia, and New Zealand. The nations with the lowest obesity rates are South Korea and Japan—each with only 3.2% of their population considered obese.

Currently, about seven percent of the world population is obese, and the number is rising.

Recent surveys show that in the United States, the rate of being overweight has doubled among children six to eleven years of age and has tripled among those twelve to seventeen years of age. Nearly 8% of children four to five years of age are overweight. Approximately 14% to 15% of all fifteen-year-olds in the United States are obese. Although 8% and 15% may not seem like particularly high percentages, when the numbers are combined for a global impact, approximately twenty-two million children under the age of five years are overweight. More specifically, among boys and girls, with regard to race and ethnicity, being overweight is the highest in Mexican American children, intermediate in African-American children, and lowest in Caucasian children. African Americans, Hispanics, Pima Indians, and other Native Americans have a particularly high predisposition to obesity.

In addition to gender, race, and ethnicity, socioeconomic and environmental factors affect the impoverished population more than the advantaged populations. For example, families in low-income areas may deal with problems of proximity to fast food restaurants, lack of access to playgrounds and fitness centers, the impact of the media, lack of affordable healthy foods, government-funded school lunches that are inadequately nourishing, and so on. These factors and their effects will be discussed in later chapters.

Obesity is not merely an inconvenience. A recent Oxford University study found that moderate obesity, which is now common, reduces life expectancy by about three years, and that severe obesity, which is less common, can shorten a person's life by ten years. This ten-year loss is equal to the effects of lifelong smoking.

One of the major concerns regarding obesity is that once you become obese, it becomes a lifelong problem. Childhood obesity is a key predictor for obesity in adulthood, so this is a problem that often does not go away. It's interesting to speculate about the impact of the family in cases of childhood obesity because, obviously, there are certain factors operating in those families but not in other families. Maybe it's lifestyle, eating habits, educational level, food addiction, or a combination of those things and some others. Genetics may play a significant role in some cases, but additional factors can "stack the deck" against a child who has the potential of becoming obese. Gender, race, ethnicity, social factors, and residential location are just some of these factors.

So, why has the rate of obesity skyrocketed so quickly? What is obesity really? How is it identified, tracked, and understood?

One explanation is that it's partially genetic. As Dr. Phyllis Speiser stated, "Obesity results from the genetic propensity to store fat in response to insulin, paired with our lifestyles with too much sedentary activity and processed energy-dense foods that have contributed to the problem of overweight."

The most basic path to obesity is that it's the result of far more energy consumed than energy utilized. Food converts to energy, which is stored in the body. If the energy is not used, fats are not being burned, and the energy is converted into fat cells.

In some cases, people are eating too many foods that are laden with excess fat and sugar. In other cases, people are inactive. All of these combined can cause obesity, but if reducing obesity were as simple as consuming fewer fats and sugar and getting active, we would probably know exactly how to fix the problem, and we would have fixed it already. Instead, there is much more to it.

A plethora of studies show the importance of the family environment in contributing to the increasing prevalence of obesity, specifically increases in food supply and caloric intake accompanied by diminishing levels of physical activity. These family studies provide strong evidence for the genetic contribution to obesity. Although it's incorrect to put all the blame for obesity on the family, the family is certainly a contributor to the global problem. In addition, a number of other factors should be considered in understanding how this problem has become so large. Specifically, it's vital to look at the effects of the public schools, the media, and poverty.

Some people like to classify problems with humans as either problems of nature or problems of nurture. But research seems to show that there is a combination of nature and nurture that can lead to obesity. Most progressive researchers and analysts know that you simply cannot have one without the other, so it's essential to look at both sides.

Despite a genetic predisposition to obesity, you still have choices, you can defy genetics, and you can choose not to let this predisposition rule your life. This is where nurture can be used to your advantage. You can increase your Health Intelligence, you can grow wiser about what kind of lifestyle you choose, and you can counter that predisposition in with positive action. Even if you have been obese or overweight, you can change with a boost to your Health Intelligence and a new, nurturing direction.

An Index of Clarification

What's the difference between overweight and obese? The categories of weight are based on your body mass index (BMI), which is a measure of your weight in relation to your height. It's easy to do. A simple calculation of your BMI would look like this for an individual who weighs two hundred pounds: BMI equals a person's weight in pounds divided by their height in inches squared, multiplied by 703. For example, for someone who is six feet tall (72") and weighs 200 pounds, the calculation would be 200 divided by 5,184 (72" X 72") multiplied by 703 = 27.12 BMI.

When you find your BMI, you can compare the number to the following categories.

Body Mass Index	
Underweight	below 18.5
Normal weight	18.5-24.9
Overweight	25.0-29.9
Obesity: Class 1	30.0-39.9
Extreme obesity	40 and up

If you find yourself in the overweight, obese, or extremely obese category, then you will benefit from some significant modifications in your lifestyle, eating habits, and health-related behaviors. This book is designed to give you valuable tools to begin the journey toward better health. If you are a parent, a loved one, a relative, or a friend of someone in the overweight or obese categories, you can benefit from the same kinds of adjustments to your lifestyle. An overweight or obese child especially needs your guidance, and you have a responsibility to provide it. You can pass on the wisdom you take from this book to anyone who may benefit from it. Becoming health intelligent is a gift that you can freely share with others.

If you're in the normal weight range, according to the above chart, you may still want to consider revising some of your lifestyle choices. As you may know, as we age our bodies do not keep the same metabolism. Throughout my childhood and even after I had my third child, I was fortunate to be able to eat what I wanted and maintain a normal weight. However, after I had my fourth child, I was already in my late thirties, and it became much harder to control my weight. I had to make a conscious effort by watching what I ate and becoming less sedentary. It became evident that my metabolism had slowed down. I could not cheat myself by eating foods that I knew contained high caloric content. I had to change the way I ate. I also had to find new ways to stay active. Although my work as a school administrator required a good deal of walking throughout the school day, it was still not enough to stabilize my weight and firm up my muscles.

Even if you are of normal weight, a change in your body chemistry may eventually impact your weight. Other variables including new restaurants popping up everywhere, new culinary delights and ghastly concoctions (for example, chocolate-covered bacon and steak dipped in butter), more on-the-go eating, and less time to be physically active can also present a challenge to your diet. Therefore, even if you are of normal weight, you can always be a little healthier and a little wiser about what you choose to consume.

For the underweight group, this could be your opportunity to learn what you may not be doing right for your body. Your body needs certain combinations of nutrients, vitamins, and minerals, and if you do not consume what's needed, you could be underweight and unhealthy in a variety of ways. This is not to say that being underweight is itself unhealthy, but there is certainly a risk associated with being outside the normal ranges. If nothing else, you may gain a little insight into your lifestyle, why you eat the way you eat, how you have changed your habits over the years, and how healthy you actually are.

Needless to say, everyone can benefit from becoming a bit more health intelligent. Nobody could possibly know all there is to know about health and food. The science is constantly changing, research is bringing in new facts on what's healthy, and the field of personal health does not remain static over time. This means that in order to be as health intelligent as possible everyone should keep abreast of the current news and research. Just like anything else, it takes time and a commitment to learn and then grow from what you learn. It can be done.

Comorbidity

Now that we have identified the weight categories and we understand that everyone can benefit from a little more knowledge about health, it might be beneficial to know exactly why we should improve our Health Intelligence. We all know, or should know, the basic, most common problems associated with being overweight or obese. Diabetes, high blood pressure, heart attacks, various cancers, knee problems, eye problems, asthma and other breathing problems are just a few of the many health effects caused by overeating, extra body weight, and obesity. The problem is that these diseases do not usually happen in isolation from one another; it's not as if we just have one issue that requires attention. People with extra weight are often overloaded with physical problems because of the weight. They may suffer from comorbidities, a combination of symptoms and illnesses that require ongoing treatment. Without proper nutrition and physical exercise, the symptoms worsen, and additional problems can set in. When your knees hurt, you do not move as easily. When you do not move as easily, exercise becomes a chore that results in pain and stress on the heart. A lack of movement leads to the desire for a more sedentary lifestyle and the chances of becoming even more overweight. The effects snowball and the problems eventually become chronic.

The comorbidities associated with obesity are problematic on their own, but many of them can also lead to more serious health problems. Childhood obesity can be accompanied by significant comorbidities and health problems that are similar to those of obese adults. Obese children often grow up to be obese adults, but in certain cases the adult problems become issues for children very early in life. Undoubtedly, these children were at risk from the start. Doctors who practice general medicine and pediatricians are finding that they are treating young children for diseases such as Type 2 diabetes that have historically been considered adult problems.

With all these problems it's no wonder that people are struggling with the higher costs of health insurance and doctor bills. Physical problems often require ongoing attention. Treatment takes time and money. For people who cannot afford medical treatment, the government and other agencies are able to step in and provide assistance. Although specifics about health insurance coverage and medical expenses are beyond the scope of this book, it's worthwhile to remember that in the United States about $150 billion per year is spent on medical costs, much of which is associated with obesity.

Regardless of the effects of the larger institutions, individuals still have choices and responsibilities in making healthy choices. But when people are consistently exposed to high fat diets, sugars, processed foods, fast foods, artificial sweeteners, caffeine, and other ingredients that have negative effects, it's extremely difficult to make appropriate choices. By the same token, when young children learn how to eat and what to eat from their parents whose choices have been limited by their circumstances, those children will follow the same unhealthy eating patterns. It becomes a vicious cycle that is terribly hard to reverse or break.

Both individuals who are obese and those who are not may find it easy to blame obesity on genetics, but there are obviously a number of other factors that must be considered. The following chapter outlines the biggest contributors to the obesity epidemic.

Individual Effects

When it comes to individual food choices, much of the responsibility is left to the individual. For example, if you're a single adult, it's likely that you choose foods that are easy to prepare and are sold in single-serving portion sizes. Even in the rare case that you are a foodie and enjoy dining out with friends or cooking at home, much of the diet of a single adult probably leaves something to be desired. Your choices include healthy options, but those are not always as easy or as filling as the not-so-healthy alternatives. For some people, being busy, being lazy, and wanting to save money become the daily eating decision makers. Fast food is both easy and affordable.

Additionally, many individuals are predisposed to unhealthy eating habits. This kind of training likely started in childhood and continued into adulthood. Perhaps your mom served heavy meals with meat and potatoes and biscuits or rolls with tons of butter-filled gravy. If you grew up on those kinds of meals, your body has been trained to expect rich, satisfying food. If you were the parent who cooked that way, you probably still cook that way; it's a hard habit to break. For a parent who thrives on being able to nourish her family with filling foods, it's an even harder habit to break. That parent's sole purpose in life is to feed and care for her family. Her way of showing love is through food. If you, as the child, love your mother, then you'll eat what is offered to you. How can you possibly say no to your own mother? It becomes a tricky, slippery slope of depending on food to foster the relationship that has always been special and rewarding. It's exceedingly hard to change that mentality. How do you make the relationship *not* about food when it has always been that way? How can mom care for you without food? How can you validate her care without eating the heavy meals on which you grew up?

But what about the child who grows up in a home where he or she is not taught to eat well? What if that child is a victim of the fast food diet or fast prep foods at home night after night? Many parents have not learned the basics of healthy eating, and if they have, it's not always easy to follow them. So their children learn by example. Those parents show their children that fast food is okay, processed foods are easy to prepare, diet sodas are the drink of choice on a daily basis, and large portions will fill you up if you're not sure where your next meal is coming from. Children will accept these habits and behaviors and will often carry them into adulthood.

Children have limited options in choosing what they eat; they are still subject to the choices of adults at home and at school. Even if they are offered healthy choices, it does not mean that they will eat what is placed before them. In my experience, many children choose not to eat certain vegetables or fruits that are offered to them, and much of the healthy food is wasted. This is especially true if these children were not exposed to these fruits and vegetables at a very early age. However, regardless of one's age, there is always some choice about what to eat and what not to eat.

Mental Health

Although the physical problems associated with obesity are often center stage in evaluation and treatment, there is no question that mental health concerns are just as important. It must be noted that mental health may require a separate course of treatment, especially in children. In addition to medical issues, obese children can have a range of psychological and behavioral problems. Psychological problems associated with childhood obesity include negative self-esteem, withdrawal from interaction with peers, depression, anxiety, and the feeling of chronic rejection.

Among severely obese adolescents, current research suggests that 48% have moderate to severe depressive symptoms, and 35% report high levels of anxiety. These percentages are alarming, especially as these numbers do not include the populations that have comorbid psychological conditions. Depressive symptoms do not necessarily lead to suicidal thoughts or attempts, but the risk is certainly there and is very real. Anxiety can include symptoms of obsessive compulsive disorder, generalized anxiety, and a myriad of other anxiety-related issues that can dramatically interfere with normal functioning.

This is the short list of common and potential mental health concerns associated with obesity in children. It would be wise to remember that these numbers and statistics do not include the list of issues that a child faces every day by virtue of just being a kid and navigating through life. Children are learning new things, making new friends, and experiencing the influence and pressures of their peer group. A child with normal weight faces numerous problems with everyday things, but an obese child faces all those problems plus the health and mental health issues resulting from being overweight. To a young child, some of those issues can seem insurmountable. Children can also have learning problems, family problems, bullying challenges, or other health issues that may be unrelated to weight. For the overweight or obese child, life can be extremely difficult. Add on all the other potential problems and that child may need a great deal of support and guidance just to survive.

These statistics are problematic on many levels, including individual and societal levels. We might look at someone we know who is overweight and decide that it's not our problem; it's an individual problem that is to be addressed by that person. Sure, we could do that, or we could decide that the obesity phenomenon is actually something we should all be worried about. After all, most of us will experience a change in our metabolism at some point, and if we are not careful obesity could become an issue. However, even if you don't become obese, you may have to deal with the related health problems of unhealthy eating and poor nutrition. So if you believe that you are not responsible for helping to improve the health of your fellow Americans, think again—we need you. We need everyone to make an effort to improve individual, family, and public health. It begins with awareness and an acceptance of the fact that we are all in this together and we can make it better. That is, if we choose to.

Despite what people might say or think, it's possible to make changes. It may be difficult, it may take time, and it may not be your favorite thing to do, but altering your lifestyle can have a monumental impact on you, your family, the children in your life, and on others whom you do not even know you have an impact.

Most of us are born with the intelligence necessary to understand the difference between healthy choices and unhealthy choices, categories of foods, basic facts about nutrition, and so forth. Most of us learn that an apple is a better health choice than a serving of pastry laden with sugar. This kind of information is not rocket science. We have learned since we were children that fruits and vegetables are good, water is necessary, and a well-rounded diet is best. Despite our intellectual understanding of what's good for us, we act emotionally. We indulge in processed foods and snacks. We've learned that fast food tastes yummy and is comparatively cheap, and that large portions are preferred because we want to get our money's worth at whatever restaurant we visit.

So despite the fact that we might *know* what is best for our bodies, we may not always *choose* that route. In fact, we have been so bombarded by images of delicious foods and ridiculous portions that we have learned to accept indulgence as a way of life. It has become an addiction. It's hard to say no.

By the same token, we have also learned that calories quickly add up and affect our bodies in ways that we dislike. We have learned that there are many different kinds of low-fat foods and sugar-free alternatives that we can try. We might have learned that some diets work better than others or that diets do not seem to work at all. We've grown accustomed to eating more than we should because it looks so yummy, because that is how our minds have been trained to understand portions, or just because it's there. Or perhaps we eat because we're not actually paying attention to what's on the plate—we're too busy watching television, chasing the children around, or driving to the next appointment. We're not being mindful of what we consume, and so our waistlines expand, our appetites double or triple, and we become more likely to overindulge because we don't even notice that we've eaten the whole thing.

Whatever the individual reasons for poor choices with regard to health and lifestyle, the issue has become global. Even if you're happy with your weight, eating habits, and health, it's likely that you could do even better. It's possible that you could feel better with just a few small changes to your daily activities. Whether you believe it or not, your choices affect others; and if you have children of your own or children who look up to you, your health behaviors can have a tremendous impact. It only makes sense to learn how you could improve your Health Intelligence.

Chapter 6

We Eat What We Learn

We are what we repeatedly do.
Excellence, then, is not an act, but a habit.
— Aristotle

In humans, Health Intelligence is rarely innate. It's a behavior that must be learned. Therefore, to discuss how Health Intelligence is learned, we need to spend a few minutes revealing the nature of learning itself.

There are three significant research paradigms offering perspectives on learning; these are the Behaviorist, Cognitivist, and Constructivist paradigms. Simply put, Behaviorists look at learning as an aspect of conditioning related to a system of rewards and targets in education. Cognitivists believe that the definition of learning as a change in behavior is too narrow and prefer to study the learner rather than his or her environment, and in particular the complexities of human memory. Constructivists believe that a learner's ability to learn relies to a large extent on what he or she already knows and understands, and that the acquisition of knowledge should be an individually tailored process of construction.

One of the earliest notions about learning was offered by the

Behaviorists. For them, learning was defined as an observable change in behavior. Behaviorists also agree that reinforcement can increase the likelihood of a behavior recurring, whereas punishment might decrease that likelihood. For example, soon after birth, a baby gets hungry and cries for something to eat. Once the bottle or the mother's breast is introduced to the child as the mode by which food is given, the baby responds automatically to that source of food every time that it's introduced. After a few months when the mother desires to wean the child from the breast or the bottle, she will gradually lessen her response to the child's cries for feeding with the breast or bottle and instead introduce a fork or spoon with solid food. Over time, the child will no longer associate feeding time exclusively with the breast or bottle, but will become increasingly more open to other food sources. This process involves little mental processing of information.

Although Behaviorist ideas served as a way to explain early learning, later theorists and researchers believed that there was much more to the process of learning than simple behavioral reactions. There was a cognitive element that had to be considered as a critical piece in the learning process.

In the 1960s, Swiss biologist and child psychologist Jean Piaget took the ideas of behaviorism and advanced the way that people think about learning and development. Piaget was one of the first researchers to develop a theory about how young children learn based on observations of his children and others. His understanding of child development was that *development precedes learning*; children must be prepared physically and mentally for new information in order to process it correctly.

Piaget suggested that intelligence is a form of adaptation—that is, being able to change and grow within a dynamic environment. He believed that children construct their own knowledge, assimilating and accommodating to the world around them by interacting with others and the environment. A child takes the information and organizes it according to what he or she already knows to improve understanding. This defines the process of learning.

Soviet psychologist Lev Semyonovich Vygotsky added a dimension of learning that included the social environment, suggesting that social interaction plays a fundamental role in cognitive development. Vygotsky theorized that social learning happens before development and stated, "Every function in the child's cultural development appears twice: first, on the social level, and later, on the individual level; first, between people (interpsychological) and then inside the child (intrapsychological)."

A review of the existing research on intelligence and early learning reveals that childhood learning stems from a combination of internal mechanisms and external environmental factors. It's no longer a question of nature versus nurture, but rather a question of how nature and nurture interact to affect learning and development.

Kids Observe and Mimic

Research suggests that children learn behavior from their environment through the process of observation. Children take their observations and internalize the activities, habits, vocabulary, and ideas of the members of the community in which they grow up.

As we know, the effect of parents on development can be immensely significant. From the very beginning of their lives and throughout childhood parents interact with their children. It's through these interactions that children acquire the behaviors that enable them to become effective members of society.

Parents are not the only ones who have an impact on a young person's life. Any individual who is observed can be considered a *model.* Children are surrounded by influential models including siblings, neighborhood children, famous athletes and movie stars, characters on TV, friends within their peer group, and teachers at school. We know that these models can be exceedingly important. The models are not always positive role models; children are also highly influenced by negative examples of behavior (for example, smoking, drinking, drug abuse, and fighting).

Children see a model and attempt to imitate the model. When the observed behaviors, values, beliefs, and attitudes of the model are incorporated into the individual's life, the process of identification is complete. Often the role model is a real person, and we hope that children will emulate only the positive behaviors. In spite of our hopes and encouragement, however, we know that children also mimic negative behaviors such as swearing, smoking cigarettes, and eating poor quality food. It's then the job of the adult to expose children to positive role models and to educate them about the potential harm in observing and mimicking negative role models.

Through positive reinforcement for appropriate mimicry and consistent assignment of consequences for emulation of negative behaviors, children can be taught the benefits and consequences of certain behaviors. When a child learns a behavior and exhibits the behavior in the presence of significant others, it's crucial for the parent, teacher, other adult, or peer to respond to the new behavior with either positive reinforcement or a consequence.

Reinforcement is meant to increase the likelihood that a

behavior will happen again. It can be external or internal. The type of reinforcement, its frequency, and its proximity to the behavior will determine whether or not the behavior continues. Reinforcement can include things such as positive verbal feedback, a toy, a sticker, a treat, a special outing, or positive feelings directed towards the young child. In addition, kids can experience vicarious reinforcement, which means he or she is learning from observing the reinforcement or consequence of someone else. For example, if one child is praised for trying a vegetable, a sibling may be willing to taste the vegetable as well in order to obtain the same kind of positive parental feedback.

Learning requires children to observe, to pay attention, to understand, to set goals, and to assume responsibility for their own learning. To help our kids learn, we must interact, activate prior knowledge, strategize, organize, and apply the new information. It's a dynamic process that requires motivation and effort.

Here are eight components that are necessary for teaching—and learning—to be successful: (1) Active involvement with the teacher, (2) Social participation, (3) Meaningful activities, (4) Relating the new information to prior knowledge, (5) Engaging in self-regulation and being reflective, (6) Aiming toward understanding rather than memorization, (7) Taking time to practice, and (8) Exploring developmental and individual differences.

There are many theories of learning, and we don't need to discuss all of them! What we can agree on is that learning is a combination of complex processes and influences. For each individual the learning process is unique and is affected by the environment. Kids learn from peers, family, media, schools, reinforcements, consequences, and internal processes that help the child learn valuable information. Learning is not an effortless process that starts and stops with the acquisition of information. Instead, learning is the result of observing, attending, practicing, and exhibiting a change in behavior based on a series of mental processes.

Dimensions of Understanding

Learning is not a simple linear or one-dimensional process. Within the complicated structure of the learning process, there are multiple dimensions of understanding.

At one end of the spectrum, there is informational learning—memorizing and recalling basic information (such as phone numbers, facts, and personal data). At the other end of the spectrum is creative learning, where individuals bring all sorts of information together in a high-level display of knowledge (for example, writing a story, drawing, or creating a business plan). In between, there are a variety of other learning levels and thinking skills that we use in tasks we encounter every day. For example, driving a car requires a set of higher level thinking skills, whereas filling out a form simply requires remembering information.

In 1956, psychologist Benjamin Bloom developed a set of levels of understanding, which is represented as a pyramid with the most complex (higher order thinking skills) at the top (see Figure 1).

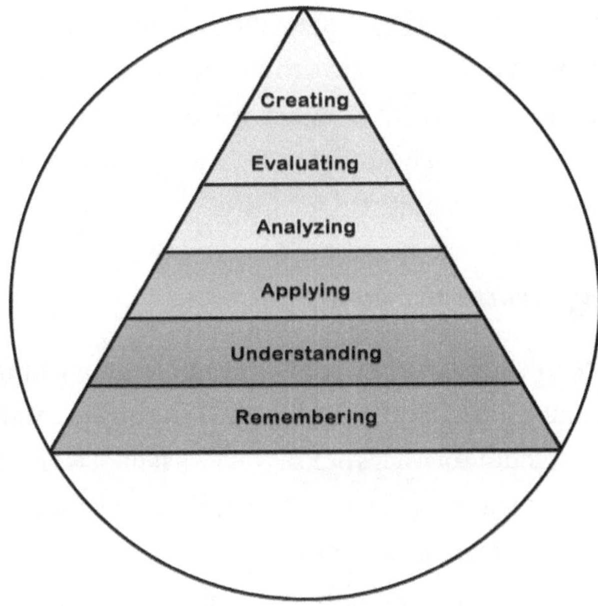

Figure 1 Bloom's Taxonomy Levels of Understanding

To help children learn we should help them to focus on a variety of different skills and levels of understanding. Providing children with a well-rounded skill set helps them apply what they have learned in new ways. Rather than just being able to recall information, children will be able to understand content in a deeper way. This will encourage them to think abstractly and make sense of information in their own way.

Critical thinking and creative thinking are at the top level, and they include skills such as comparison, classification, sequencing, cause and effect, patterning, webbing, analogies, deductive and inductive reasoning, forecasting, planning, hypothesizing, and critiquing. Creative thinking involves creating something new or original. It involves the skills of flexibility, originality, fluency, elaboration, brainstorming, modification, imagery, associative thinking, attribute listing, metaphorical thinking, and forced relationships. The aim of creative thinking is to stimulate curiosity and promote divergence. Another pictorial representation of Bloom's taxonomy can be found in Figure 2, which outlines basic skills in each of the cognitive domains.

Learning Health Behavior

What does this mean for the development of better eating habits and the acquisition of Health Intelligence? Starting in childhood, a basic understanding of what's healthy and what's not is vital to every individual. Remembering and understanding food categories such as fruits and vegetables is also essential. Even more importantly, health information is constantly evolving, and the wealth of new content requires us to apply, synthesize, analyze, and evaluate the information in new ways. We must use higher order thinking skills to process the changing information. If we're not accustomed to using those kinds of skills, we need to practice. We also know that learning results from a combination of nature and nurture. We need to understand better how genetics impact health and eating so that we can provide the best environment for ourselves and our family.

Learning Health Behavior

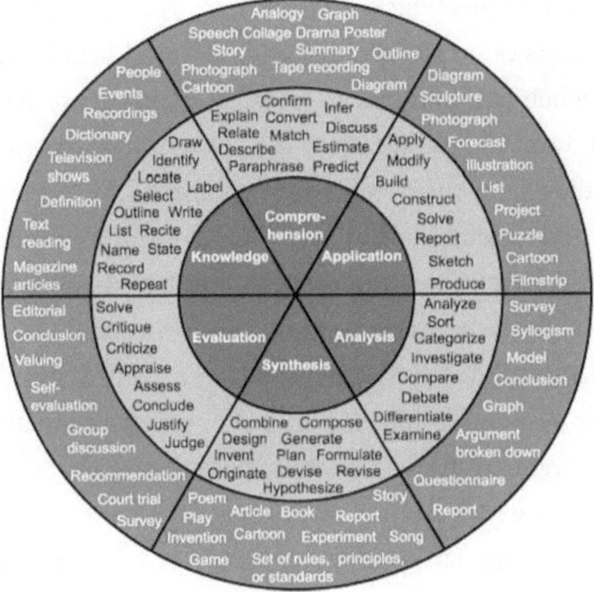

Figure 2. Bloom's taxonomy of learning.

We know that genetics play a role in obesity, and we know that the same is true of environmental factors. We need to look at how the two interact to exacerbate childhood obesity. It's clear that children learn from others and the environment around them, so it's no surprise that this is how eating behaviors are learned. Children are influenced by what others are eating: they learn through exposure, social learning, and associative learning.

The family environment can interact with genetic predispositions to produce patterns of food preferences, food consumption, and physical activity, which in turn can lead to childhood obesity. The social context in which children's eating patterns develop is important because the eating behavior of people in that environment serves as a model for the developing child. Studies suggest that modeling by an older child, a friend, or a fictional hero can impact a child's food preferences.

Parents often assume that children need help in determining what, when, and how much to eat. It makes sense. Most parents do not want their children to eat potato chips and candy all day long; they want their children to choose healthy options such as fruits and vegetables. But imposing consumption practices that restrict eating or set unreasonable limitations on types of food means children have fewer opportunities to learn about self-control. When a child's food consumption is restricted, that child does not learn to respond to internal cues of hunger and satiety. Similarly, when parents restrict access to certain foods, it may enhance the child's liking for that food and can increase desire for intake.

Restricting children's consumption of "bad" foods and encouraging consumption of "good" foods does not actually work in the way that parents intend it to. Instead of encouraging healthy eating, such restrictions send the child mixed messages. The child may view the eating of vegetables and fruits or other healthy choices as a negative experience, counteracting the parents' attempts to encourage healthy eating for the sake of healthy eating. Instead of liking healthy foods because they taste delicious, children might feel punished when required to eat certain foods (for example, vegetables or fruits) just to acquire a preferred food (for example, more noodles, bread, or dessert).

Mixed messages about food often do not end with everyday rituals around the table. Most of the forbidden or restricted foods are the same ones that are typically offered at positive social events such as parties, dinners out, and holiday celebrations. Children learn that such foods are positive in some instances but not in others. Why is that okay? It certainly is confusing.

The solution is to offer the child *a range of acceptable options* from which the child can choose, including how much to consume.

Parents as Models

It's no surprise that parents have a particularly influential role in their children's lives. Parents shape their children's eating environments in a variety of ways. From the early decision about an infant's feeding method, to the foods they make available and accessible to children, to direct modeling influences, to limiting (or failing to limit) media exposure in the home, to the way they interact with children in the eating context, parents can have a tremendous and ongoing impact on their children's daily eating behavior. It makes sense that what parents eat, children eat. Children observe their parents and are likely to adopt their food selection patterns and eating behavior.

Parents' eating behaviors and attitudes closely correspond to those of their children. Studies have confirmed that the diets of parents and their children tend to be very similar, and indicate a strong association between a parent's and child's snack food intake for all kinds of snacks, not just the unhealthy type. This kind of information provides support for the social learning theory that features the idea of modeling; and as any grandmother knows, children's diets are affected by the types of food eaten by their parents.

Parents expose their children to a variety of foods every day in what they eat and what they serve in the home, as well as what they eat when they dine out. Mere exposure—the extent to which fruits and vegetables are made available and accessible to children—can shape what kinds of foods a child eats and chooses to eat. Exposure to new foods can change intake and preferences because children grow to like and eat what is familiar, and familiar foods are those that are present in the environment. Repeated experience with tasty foods, such as high-energy foods, can enhance children's preferences for those foods via associative conditioning, and children will begin to include those foods in their diet. Maybe a child does not like cauliflower the first time he or she eats it, but, with repeated exposure and new preparations, the child may grow to like cauliflower. It's possible. If a child is exposed to new choices and new recipes, and is encouraged to sample while observing a parent enjoying that same food, learning new eating behaviors can become a positive experience.

Anyone who has watched the Food Network knows that children of one culture will happily eat foods that children in another culture find revolting. Fried grasshopper, anyone? It's all a matter of cultural conditioning.

Patterns of eating in a household can be influenced by factors such as availability, accessibility, and children's food preferences. For example, childrens' preferences for high-fat foods predict their fat consumption; these preferences in turn are related to their parents' weight control problems. If a parent chooses to eat PopTarts for breakfast, the child will learn that it's an acceptable choice. If parents choose to eat on the run (or while moving around the kitchen) most days, the child will develop eating patterns that do not include relaxing at a table with family and taking time to enjoy the meal. If a parent does not place priority on obtaining fresh fruits and vegetables but chooses prepared, frozen meals or processed foods, the child will likely choose that pattern as well.

Parents exhibit eating patterns all the time: eating in front of the television, finishing the entire bag of chips, eating sugary foods for breakfast, eating late night snacks, over consuming when eating out, and so on. Meanwhile, children watch every move their parents make and model their eating behavior after that of their parents. Common sense suggests that educating parents about what to feed their children is critical; however, it's equally crucial for parents to modify their own diets in order to provide a more positive model for young children to imitate.

In short, talk is cheap; to get results parents must walk the walk. You cannot tell your kids to lay off the Twinkies when you've got one stuffed in your own mouth.

Chapter 7

Seefood – We Eat What We See

To keep the body in good health is a duty,
otherwise we shall not be able to keep our mind
strong and clear.
— Buddha

There are thousands of fast food restaurants in the world—McDonald's, Burger King, Wendy's, Taco Bell, Sonic, KFC, Rally's, and many more—serving just about any kind of food you can imagine. Fast food has, of course, been under scrutiny for many years for being less than healthy. Sure, the food is reasonably affordable, but the caloric intake is excessive, and fast food has taken a toll on public health. Children are at high risk of being consistent consumers because of advertising ploys, addictive food, toys or prizes with meals, and so on.

Everyone probably has some sort of story associated with McDonald's or any of the other fast food joints. Beyond the food, there's something about the memory of a time at that restaurant. For some people, visiting McDonald's has become a family tradition;

maybe when you were little grandpa took you there for a shake and some fries, or maybe it was the place you stopped when you were on that family vacation and everyone got hungry. It was there at every rest stop, it was fast, it was easy, and everyone was able to find something he or she liked on the menu.

Nowadays there's somewhere to eat on almost every corner of every town. You can count on fast food to be there, and you can count on fast food to be generally consistent, taste good, and be affordable. People like that kind of predictability. People like knowing what to expect (those generously salted fries, just the right amount of ketchup and onions, two pickles, and a shake with the perfect thickness). How disappointed are you when you get that one soggy fry? It's almost not worth the dollar you paid for it if it's not just like every other time you have purchased it. This is conveyer belt food. You should get what you expect.

It's difficult to mass-produce food of any sort of quality, so these restaurants end up being subpar in terms of nutrition. Research suggests that children who frequently eat fast food consume more total energy, more energy per gram of food, more total fat, more total carbohydrates, more added sugars, less fiber, less milk (calcium), and fewer fruits and vegetables than children who eat fast food infrequently. Of course, we all know that burgers and fries are high in calories, and places such as McDonald's have frequently been criticized for offering high-fat, calorie-dense meals, and for creating advertising campaigns geared toward children.

In response, McDonald's has started offering choices with kids' meals; you can order milk instead of soda pop, and you can choose apples instead of French fries. But if you're like most kids, I'm guessing you'll probably choose the fries. The fries are yummy.

There's no denying that. They are addictive, warm, and satisfying. Kids love potatoes; they are safe, tasty, and reliable. As a child, if I had to choose between fries or apples, I'm pretty sure that most times I would have chosen fries, especially if the importance of choosing the apple was not explained. You can instruct your child to choose apples, but that may not always work when a more appealing option is available. So, despite the restaurants' attempts to offer healthy options such as salads and yogurt parfaits, my guess is that most people do not choose them. When you're standing in front of the kid at the counter with the paper hat and you're watching the girl in the back dump the hot fries into the bin and salt them with that powdery salt, you are already in a sensory coma from the variety of fast food aromas—and you're going to choose the fries. It's for you to find the strength to make that healthy choice.

Children usually have some choices, but parents have more. No parent is forced to enter a fast food restaurant. Rather than fighting the institution that is fast food, purchase your own food and cook it at home. I know some people do not have the time, do not know how to cook, or have a million other excuses, but if you know that fast food is not healthy, then for goodness sakes make your own! As a matter of fact, you can make a really decent burger for a truly affordable price if you actually tried to. We do not have to eat what restaurants offer. We can choose not to.

If we do choose to eat it, it's important to be well informed about the potential consequences of our actions. McDonald's is now disclosing the calorie counts of their menu items. But I can assure you that if the customers do not become Health Intelligent, the eating habits of most individuals will not change. They are hooked and have fallen prey to the juicy burgers and fatty fries. Making that kind of educated decision is necessary in most venues, and it's certainly no different in the case of what you choose to put into your body.

So how do we know what we're putting in our bodies? We can read food labels and we can do as little or as much research as we choose until we feel comfortable with what we're eating. It's not hard to find the nutritional content of most foods, including those that are served at fast food restaurants. Nutritional content—calories, grams of fat, and all kinds of other information about fast food meals, sides, and beverages—is published online and posted in the restaurants. You just have to ask or seek it out on your own. It's like learning about a medicine before you take it; it's a good idea to know the side effects and potential hazards of anything you consume.

In their groundbreaking report "Evaluating Fast Food Nutrition and Marketing to Youth," researchers Jennifer Harris, Marlene Schwartz, and Kelly Brownell investigated the healthfulness of fast food meals. They found some alarming numbers. For example, only twelve of 3,039 possible kids' meal combinations meet nutrition criteria for preschoolers. Only fifteen meet nutrition criteria for older children. Beyond the lack of nutritional value, they also found higher sugar and fat content. Teens between the ages of thirteen and seventeen consume 800 to 1,200 calories in an average fast food meal, including 30% or more calories from sugar and saturated fat. Young people can consume *half* of their maximum daily recommended sodium intake in just *one meal* at a fast food restaurant.

Fast food marketing has always targeted the youth, but with the rise in websites, social networks, and other digital media, the tween and teen audiences have become even more prone to the ill effects of marketing.

Young children are increasingly exposed to this kind of

marketing. Through websites such as McDonald's Ronald.com, internet-based marketing targets kids as young as age two years. As if one website were not enough, McDonald's actually has thirteen different websites that get 365,000 unique child visitors and 294,000 unique teen visitors each month.

The Fast Food and Media Crossover

Fast food companies are using increasingly sophisticated marketing campaigns that penetrate many areas of a potential consumer's everyday life experience. McDonald's and Burger King have created sophisticated advertising games and virtual worlds (for example, McWorld.com, HappyMeal.com, and ClubBK.com) that are designed to engage children and build brand loyalty. Nine restaurant Facebook pages had more than a million fans. Eight of the fast food chains have Smartphone apps to reach young consumers anytime, anywhere. Obviously, technology has helped widen the fast food consumer base, and there is tremendous potential for future advertising to reach even more children, tweens, and teens. All demographics are targets through digital media and technology, and those avenues are likely to continue to grow and expand. Fast food is not going away anytime soon. That's okay. It's actually nice to have that available to you when you need it. But the point is that consumers must educate themselves on the choices they have, and fast food restaurants must find ways of making and serving healthier foods.

Just because it's there, and sales gurus are making it easier and easier to access, does not mean we have to consume it. We still have choices. We always have choices. It's essential to educate yourself about what you're eating. Then if after everything you've learned you decide that you still want to consume a juicy quarter pounder and the extra large fries with extra salt that you have added yourself, go ahead. One meal is not going to kill you. But when you make that choice, really enjoy that burger. I mean, enjoy it as if it were your last meal. Savor every last bite. Eat slowly and really taste it. Scrape that little bit of cheese off the wrapper and eat that too. When you are done, sit back and let yourself feel satisfied and full.

Being healthy is not about depriving yourself of the things you like; it's about allowing yourself to indulge in them once in a while and thoroughly enjoying them. If we deprive ourselves, we begin to think of a particular food as good or bad, and we enlist the help of shame in modifying our food choices. That's never a smart idea. We can make a less-than-healthy choice every now and then. As the old saying goes, "Everything in moderation—including moderation." When we're not deprived of something that tastes delicious, and we allow ourselves to enjoy it, then we're more likely to choose something healthy and enjoyable tasting the next time, knowing that we can indulge again when we truly want to. Nothing is forbidden. We always have choices. What is most comforting to remember is, we can choose something healthier for the next meal. It's all about balance.

I would also like to add that our taste buds grow dull if they are exposed to the same salty, oily fast foods day after day. Children who eat processed fast food on a regular basis become accustomed to it. The excessive amounts of fat and salt seem perfectly normal to them, while the clean sharp flavors of fresh foods seem alien. Parents need to tip the balance in the opposite direction. Children need to become acclimated to fresh foods and regard these as normal, and if this is accomplished, then they will consider processed fast food to be exceptional. I know of more than one kid who, having grown up eating fresh homemade foods, won't set foot in a McDonald's because they think the food is "gross." Far from regarding fast food as a treat, they regard is as something to be avoided.

How can parents tip the scales? They can do so by providing only healthy foods at home and by limiting exposure to fast food restaurants. Yes, this means saying "no" to children and enduring the occasional tantrum. But a battle now and then is a small price to pay for a lifetime of better health.

Television

People are quick to blame whatever they can for societal problems. Television has been the target of blame for many ills and is certainly a logical target of blame for the obesity epidemic. Various results from research conducted on the effects of television on childhood obesity show that television does affect children in a number of ways. Viewing of television means children are sedentary and are therefore not participating in physical activity. Decreased physical activity, along with increased calorie intake, is one of the underlying causes of obesity. When television viewing, on-demand movies, video games, and other forms of passive media are in competition with active sports and games, children are easily sucked in. In the United States, research suggests that only about 25% of adolescents report regular exercise, and an alarming 14% say they do not exercise at all. Although these figures refer to adolescents, young children are likely to have similar rates, depending on the extent of the parents' efforts to control television viewing and activity.

The challenge is not only that kids who watch television are physically inactive. Research has shown that television viewing results in increased snacking behavior. When children are focused on watching television, they are not concentrating on what they are eating. They are not eating mindfully, so their bodies do not cue the satiety reaction—they do not know they are full. Consequently the number of calories consumed is drastically increased.

Finally, watching television has been shown to interfere with normal sleep patterns, which exacerbates overall poor health with increased fatigue, increased sedentary behavior, and the consumption of more unhealthy foods to maintain energy.

Beyond the basic lack of physical activity inherent in watching television, there are numerous effects that programming and commercials can have on young children. If children watch an average of seven hours of television per day, these effects can be tremendously powerful. Children who have a television set in their bedrooms spend even more hours watching and snacking.

For every hour of kids' television, children see about eleven food advertisements. Food is the most frequently advertised product on children's television. Children can learn unhealthy behaviors from the programming as well as the relentless advertisements for unhealthy foods. The foods featured in television fiction are most often low-nutrient drinks (such as coffee, fizzy drinks, and alcohol) and snacks (primarily sweets or salty snacks).

It's easy to blame the mass media, but is the media responsible when parents allow their kids to watch endless programs, play mind-numbing video games, or use the Internet? We need to know what factors influence the acceptance or rejection of a specific message. Why do some media messages mobilize public action while others do not? Is what people bring to their understanding of stories more relevant than media coverage? Perhaps it's even relevant to question whether policy makers are simply responding to exaggerated media headlines and diverting resources from other killer diseases that are more expensive to diagnose and treat. Exploring these questions will help us understand the link between obesity and the media.

Advertising Messages

No matter where you look, advertising messages about food and eating habits are focused on a few basic concepts, including food that is quick, food that is easy to prepare, food that is personalized to individuals' tastes, and food that is available and easy to take on the go. There are now mobile apps that show you where you can order food to be delivered, how you can make recipes at home, and everything else you could ever want to know about food.

The Internet is a rich source of recipes, tips, ideas, and more—all about food. Do a quick Google search and there are 107 million web links that pop up for the latest easy-weeknight-meal ideas. Rachel Ray attracts viewers with her thirty-minute meals. Gone are the days of recipe books and recipe card boxes. Everything you could ever need is at your fingertips via the computer or your phone.

There is an increased focus on preparing meals quickly because in this fast-paced world we think that we do not have time to cook and labor over meals as previous generations might have done. We want to have food quickly after a long, difficult, busy day, and we want foods that are fast and easy to prepare. This does not mean fast food exactly. Many food companies have updated their taglines and advertising slogans to reflect this fast-paced approach to dining (for example, Tyson Chicken Wonders: the five-minute meal).

The emphasis on, and desire for, fast eating is supported by companies that market foods that are prepackaged, premixed, precooked, or ready to warm in just minutes. Beginning in the early 1940s, companies introduced a single meal on one plate that was appropriate for military or airline travel. After some modifications and evolutions in technology, Swanson created their first frozen dinners in 1954, which were eventually called TV dinners; they could be heated in minutes and could be eaten in front of the television, bringing a new audience of couch potatoes to meal time.

From breakfast to dinner and even dessert, you can choose frozen or prepared meals that fit your budget, your style, and your taste. Eggo waffles, frozen pancakes, sausage, scrambled eggs, Healthy Choice or Lean Cuisine lunches and dinners, Smart Ones, Banquet Meals, Lunchables, Swanson Dinners, and Stouffer's Dinners—all of these and many more line the shelves and fill the frozen food cases of supermarkets. These days, eating is easy. Everything is prepackaged, precooked, and ready to go. You can take it with you wherever you need to be. You do not even have to plan ahead what to make for dinner; you can just pop open the freezer and make a choice just like you would at a restaurant. You can choose from any number of different dishes and sides, a variety of ethnic meals, and endless pasta, meat, and vegetable choices. There is something for everyone: children, people with diabetes, vegetarians, people who are counting calories, and the big man who loves his meat and potatoes in large portions. It's efficient because you get an entire meal in one little box that is ready in under five minutes. All you need is a microwave. These meals are extremely portable for on-the-go consumers, which is a market demographic that continues to grow. McCormick even offers prepackaged spices to flavor your twenty-minute meal so that you get the flavor you want with little room for error.

Ore-Ida has even made it easy to have the French fries you love in the comfort of your own kitchen. Their microwaveable French fries make it possible to prepare restaurant-style fast food in minutes at home. As if it were not already easy enough, Kraft had to come out with Easy Mac. Lunchables and Uncrustables are especially designed for the mom who does not have time or does not choose to make her kids' lunches every day. What could be easier than stackable, kid-sized lunch meats and cheeses with crackers and a juice box all in one hermetically sealed container? Maybe a premade peanut butter and jelly sandwich without the crust…

Magazines and cooking websites are riddled with taglines such as Fast Food, Quick Summer Dinners, Super Simple Cooking, Fast Weeknight Menus, Time Saving Tips, Make-Ahead Meals, Healthy and Fast, Short-Cut Recipes, and 15 Easy Party Recipes. Even thirty-minute meals have been replaced with twenty-minute meals. Television's latest trend is beat-the-clock shows such as Chopped, Sweet Genius, and Cupcake Wars where competitors race to the finish. Sure, they are judged on taste, creativity, and other criteria, but the constant is the clock that they must race against.

People want food fast. They also want it easy, which goes hand in hand with fast. Companies have capitalized on the desire for ease and effortlessness with taglines such as "Lays Potato Chips—Happiness is easy," "Three basic ingredients," and "Corningware—Of all the things you will put into it, effort is not one of them."

Even if you want healthy food that is not processed, you can enter the grocery store and find prechopped onions, cabbage, lettuce, or a variety of other vegetables. You do not even have to slice your carrots anymore, and some whole vegetables are prewashed. You can find watermelon chunks, pineapple halves, and fruit that is prepared and ready to be eaten. Even the deli at your grocery stores may offer a shortcut to cold cut favorites; prepackaged sandwich turkey and cheeses are displayed in a fridge alongside the deli so you do not have to wait in line to personalize your order. Grocery stores also have the usual staples close to the checkout lines so you can quickly enter the store and grab your milk, bread, and other necessities and be back in the car in five minutes.

Advertising to Children

Advertising that is geared toward children has long been considered inappropriate and problematic for a number of reasons. Much of the advertising to American youth has been focused on food, specifically cereals, fast food, candy, carbonated drinks, high-sugar foods and drinks, snacks packed with calories, chips, cookies, and a variety of prepackaged snacks. To lure children, fast food commercials promote the idea of a free toy with the purchase of a happy meal. Cereal boxes are covered with cartoon characters, bright colors, and large, fun, child-friendly fonts.

A typical breakfast food that is marketed directly to children is Pop-Tarts. Exotic, outrageous flavors, sprinkles, frosting, and bold advertising make this an easy sell to kids. The website is designed for kids too; it's full of games, activities, puzzles, and more. Wild combinations appeal to kids who like colorful, flavorful food, and there's always a new flavor to try so kids will not get bored with the same-old, same-old every day. Pop-Tarts features Ice Cream Shoppe flavors, Gingerbread, Wildlicious flavors, Hot Fudge Sundae, Cookies and Cream, and a wide variety of other flavors that appeal to kids and adults. Add Hello Kitty or Darth Vader to the box and you can sell even more Pop-Tarts to kids.

Food and beverage companies in the United States spend more than $1.6 billion each year to attract the attention of children. Much of that money goes to licensing fees that allow the companies to put popular TV and movie characters on their packages. Characters such as SpongeBob, Dora, Shrek, and the Ninja Turtles increase sales for these companies. This is problematic because licensed characters most often turn up on junk food packaging.

You cannot tell from the wrapping, but these Snickers bars are actually filled with green-colored nougat to make them even more Shrek-like. Probably unappetizing to most adults (except my husband; he would eat a Snickers no matter what color it was), this change in packaging and product is an effort to attract a young audience. Look closely at the nutrition information and you will find that one bar has half of a child's recommended fat intake for an entire day. I do not imagine a child would stop at one quarter of the bar or even half of it once it is opened, but maybe a savvy parent will encourage the child to save some calories for another day.

Nabisco did a similar promotion geared toward young Incredible Hulk fans with the all-time favorite, Oreo, but the crème filling was not green. Still, the packaging is directed at children.

The crust of the Ninja Turtles Pudding Pie was actually dyed a delicious turtle green. The Shrek Twinkies were altered so the cream filling was colored green. Some food companies add a twist like this, but others just slap the character on the box and call it a day. Either way, children see the box, or they are drawn to the snack, which is often an unhealthy choice.

It's not uncommon to see superheroes and cartoon characters

on packaging of all kinds of food, but much of the time these child-friendly characters are featured on junk food such as cookies, popsicles, candy, bakery products, and chips. SpongeBob SquarePants Popsicles have the added visual interest of SpongeBob-related shapes like the pineapple and Patrick the Starfish inside them.

Fruit snacks are common kid-friendly treats featuring well-known kid favorites such as Tinker Bell, Snoopy, Dora, Spider-Man, Elmo, and many others. Every so often, Kellogg's and other companies will come out with fruit snacks that feature the newest kid-friendly movie characters so that there will always be a new face on the box to entice young children, girls and boys alike. To a parent, fruit snacks may seem to be a nutritious choice, especially because they claim to be made with real fruit. However, if you look at the label, the first two ingredients are corn syrup and sugar; apple puree is third. So there is actually not much real fruit in them. One pouch of fruit snacks contains eleven grams of sugar and seventy calories.

Salty snacks are just as liable to have packaging that is geared toward young children, tweens, and teens. For example, Chester the Cheetah is the cool, smooth-talking cat that sells Cheetos. He is hip and trendy, he's got attitude, and he loves cheese—at least highly processed cheese. He appeals to a young audience to the point that he has been featured on everything from a plush doll to a video game. He rhymes, he wears funky glasses, he plays sports, he rides a motorcycle, and he's made a guest appearance on *Family Guy*. He's the all around cool spokes-cat for cheesy, salted, high-calorie, high-sodium snacks.

Pringles—those space-age processed crisps in a can that vaguely resemble potato chips—used the slogan, "Once you pop, you can't stop." Pringles have only about 42% potato content, the remainder being wheat starch and flours (potato, corn, and rice) mixed with vegetable oils and an emulsifier. Pringles offers jazzy commercials with young kids eating chip after chip after chip. Flavors include kid favorites such as pizza and ranch. Interestingly, Pringles even invented the Pringles Print, which features loveable kid characters and kid-friendly text. On the website you can design your own can with Pop Art, or you can purchase a speaker to add on to your empty Pringle can. What will they think of next?

To be fair, favorite cartoon characters have been featured on packaging for fruits, vegetables, soup, raisins, juice, yogurt, oatmeal, crackers, cookies, organic products, and many more healthy choices. These attempts to combat the idea that cartoon characters sell only junk food are heartening, but it remains to be seen as to whether or not these products sell as well as the unhealthy food choices with character packaging. Once the package of fresh healthy food gets to your home, and you cook, prepare, and serve what's inside it, part of the challenge is still getting your child to eat the spinach or the green beans. Maybe the idea that SpongeBob likes broccoli will motivate a child to eat it; we know it works for junk food. We can try it and exude our enthusiasm about a super vegetable.

Some advocates of healthy eating have suggested that we ban the placement of cartoon characters on foods that are designed for children. I wonder if that's possible. Food companies are exceptionally powerful, and they have found what works to sell their products. I imagine there would be tremendous push back at any attempts to modify advertising. Americans do still believe in the ideas of free speech, branding, and limited government control over the corporate or private sector. Do we want the government putting limitations on what we see, market, value, purchase, and consume?

Chapter 8

Poverty – We Eat What We Can Afford

> Change will not come if we wait for some other person or some other time. We are the ones we've been waiting for. We are the change that we seek.
> — Barack Obama

I would like to begin this chapter by putting the discussion of today's high rates of obesity into a broader historical context.

It's generally accepted that healthy adults need between 2,000 and 2,500 calories per day. It's possible to survive on 1,500 calories per day or even less. Over the course of thousands of years of human history, through periods of feast and famine, the average person was lucky to get enough calories for optimal health and sustenance. If you were poor, you ate less. If your crops failed, you went hungry. People on the bottom of the economic ladder risked starvation. Many foods that we take for granted—animal protein, fresh fruits, sugar, spices—were treats to be enjoyed on special occasions. Well into the twentieth century, starvation, not obesity, was the most significant challenge to human existence.

During the past fifty years, in advanced industrialized countries, and with some exceptions—largely due political mismanagement, not agrarian production capacity—this has changed. There has developed an economic condition that is unprecedented in human history: we produce more food than we can eat. For example, according to a study by the University of Michigan, in 2006 the United States food industry provided 3,900 calories per person per day. Accounting for waste, the average American consumed 2,594 calories per day in 2009—an increase of twenty percent from 1970.

Today, we live in a sea of food. Few people in America are at risk of starvation. You would think that under such circumstances, the rich folks who had leisure time and vast resources would be the first to become obese. Some have. But we also see a condition that a nineteenth-century observer would have found to be utterly fantastic: people living in poverty who are obese. How is this possible? In fact, it's not just that we see poor people who happen to be obese; we see evidence that poverty is a contributing *cause* of obesity.

Despite the government's attempt at leveling the playing field with school lunches, breakfasts, and media restrictions, poverty remains one of the most important factors in the rising levels of obesity. Poverty has a significant impact on the lives of millions of people in the United States and around the world. Anyone can become poor; poverty does not discriminate on the basis of race, education level, socioeconomic status, or gender. In the aftermath of the Great Recession, the job market and the housing market remained unstable and unpredictable. Even for those who were still lucky enough to have jobs, the future was uncertain. For those who had been in poverty for some time, the future remained bleak as job opportunities vanished, the value of homes declined or stagnated, and obesity levels continued to rise.

Researchers have studied the connection between poverty and education and they have consistently found that as an individual's education level increases, so too does his or her socioeconomic level. The inverse is also true—as socioeconomic level decreases, so does the educational level. It's relatively common knowledge that children and families in poverty have fewer social, financial, physical, educational, familial, and spiritual resources. Without this type of critical social capital, families in poverty typically have lower achievement and success.

Similarly, children who grow up in poverty often receive subpar education. Without the necessary tools to advance in society, individuals who are consistently below the poverty level will likely remain in a disadvantaged position. Gaining the needed social capital to advance requires opportunity, information, support, and guidance, all of which reduced in low-income areas.

The association between poverty, lower education levels, and poorer health has been relatively stable for years but remains a concern. It makes sense that better-educated people are more likely to be employed and well-paid. They have a greater sense of control over their health and their lives, and they often have more social support. They have the social capital that is needed for social mobility.

Family income affects many aspects of a child's life, and health is no exception. Although income is strongly related to achievement, research shows that if a child from a poor family is given the same learning opportunities as a child from a more affluent family, he or she can achieve at a similar or higher level. This has been proven to be true in a number of Title 1 schools where 90% of the students qualify for free or reduced-price lunch and 90% are from ethnic groups that are in the minority of the population. In these same schools, 90% have scored well in reading and mathematics on standardized tests.

Therefore, it's not *ability* that is in question but rather *opportunity.*

Children who live in extreme poverty for many years seem to suffer the worst outcomes of any population of young children. The timing of poverty is critical for certain child outcomes. Children who live in poverty during their preschool and early school years without any intervention to foster healthy living practices will be prone to becoming unhealthy in later years.

Research has also shown a relationship among the variables of poverty, educational level, and obesity. In general, people with lower income and lower education levels are more likely to become obese than those with higher income and higher education levels. The theory behind this finding is that people who are "advantaged" by education and income may have a greater awareness of healthy habits and better access to health care, healthy foods, and fitness facilities.

People in highly educated households are less likely to be obese. The overall prevalence of obesity decreases as income and education levels increase. Although there are some differences in the obese populations under scrutiny, research has found that between 2007 and 2008 childhood obesity levels increased at all income levels, and that between 2005 and 2008 obesity increased for all education levels.

These findings suggest that something else was operating as a significant influence during the time periods examined. Was it television, advertising, school lunches, school breakfasts, or technology? It's essential to take a close look at the factors that affect obesity rates.

Childhood obesity may be associated with food insecurity—a limited or uncertain access to enough nutritious food. Parents may worry that their food resources will run out before they get the next set of food stamps or income check. They may literally not know where their next meal is coming from. Household and childhood food insecurity are associated with being at risk for overweight status and actual overweight status in many demographic categories of children, particularly in teens, females, white children, and those from families below the poverty level.

A number of social variables may increase the risk of child obesity. Specifically, families with higher household incomes have lower obesity levels; however, home ownership is paradoxically associated with an increased risk of obesity. This is pure speculation, but if you are secure in your living situation (with a permanent residence that you have invested in) perhaps you are also more likely to be secure in your food resources and, therefore, more likely to overeat or overindulge.

Children with Medicaid insurance (government-provided insurance for the poorest families) may have higher obesity risk compared with commercially insured children. Despite measures to equalize health care, the at-risk groups are still showing high levels of obesity. Why are these Medicaid clients at risk for obesity? Does this mean that government health insurance programs are inadequate? Does this mean there is not substantial health care for the poorest members of society? Does there need to be more in the way of preventative care and education on health-related issues?

Other environmental factors increase the risk for obesity, including access to healthy foods in local supermarkets, places to exercise, and neighborhood safety. On a level that extends beyond the child's home and immediate social environment, general social disadvantage creates an inherent risk of obesity. Whether or not people accept it, families in poverty have tremendous disadvantages on a variety of different levels. It's clear that multiple factors can impact physical health. You might say the chips are stacked against poor people when it comes to obesity. This is not to say that people cannot counteract these factors, but the obstacles are certainly there.

School Lunches

In an effort to combat the effects of poverty and low income on eating habits, in 1946 the U.S. government instituted the National School Lunch Act. Each federally funded program is overseen by the Food and Nutrition Service of the U.S. Department of Agriculture (USDA) but administered by state education agencies. Schools deciding to participate in the programs must offer meals that meet federal nutritional requirements.

In 1995, after research showed that many school lunches failed to meet nutrition requirements, Congress passed the School Meals Initiative for Healthy Children, a program that included school breakfast and lunch programs for children in public schools. Research on the school lunch program since 1995 has shown that almost two thirds of school children eat a National School Lunch

Program lunch and consume about one third of their total calories from this meal.

The National School Lunch Program provides lunch to over 29 million children each school day, covering approximately 99,000 schools (95% of all public and private schools) with 17.5 million students receiving reduced-price or free meals. The largest populations of children who receive these meals include low-income, African American, and Hispanic children.

Unfortunately, school lunch program lunches often fail to meet nutrition requirements and have an especially high fat content. Children receiving free or reduced-price school lunches through the National School Lunch Program tend to have worse health outcomes on average than observationally similar children who do not participate, especially in the case of food insecurity.

School Breakfast Program

The federal School Breakfast Program (SBP) was first established in 1966 as a two-year pilot project designed to provide categorical grants to assist schools serving breakfasts to "nutritionally needy" children. In 1975, the program was made permanent by subsequent amendments. During the 2005-2006 school year, the program provided breakfast to roughly 9.6 million children in 82,000 schools with 7.7 million children receiving reduced-price or free breakfasts.

Despite the lack of positive effects associated with the National School Lunch Program, the breakfast program shows more hope, more positive outcomes, and more benefits to the child consumer. While some research has suggested that participation in the National School Lunch Program actually exacerbates the current epidemic of obesity, the School Breakfast Program has been called a valuable tool in the current battle against childhood obesity, because participation in at the kindergarten level is associated with a greater change in child weight between kindergarten and third grade for many children.

Meals must meet requirements for health from the USDA. For breakfast, this entails no more than 30% of calories derived from fat and less than 10% from saturated fat. Breakfasts also must provide one fourth of the recommended dietary allowance (RDA) for protein, calcium, iron, Vitamin A, and Vitamin C, and contain an age-appropriate level of calories. For lunches, the same restrictions on fat apply. However, lunches must provide one third of the RDA for protein, calcium, iron, Vitamin A, Vitamin C, and an age-appropriate level of calories. In addition, all meals are recommended to contain reduced levels of sodium and cholesterol and to increase the level of dietary fiber.

Vending Machines

In addition to providing government-funded breakfasts and lunches, schools were asked by school district authorities to restrict from vending machines and menus foods of minimal nutritional value such as soda. In January 2002, Oakland, California, was the first major school district to ban junk food in vending machines, a step which cost them an estimated $650,000 in lost revenues annually. Although this is a large amount of money, the potential effects on health and education are immeasurable.

Consumption of regular sodas and other soft drinks has shown a steady decline in schools across the country. Studies have reported that in 2004 students were drinking 12.5 ounces of soda per week, whereas in 2009, they were drinking only 0.5 ounces. There has also been a steady drop in sugar consumption from sugary snacks, which has decreased by fourteen percent over that same time period. Although the complete banning of sugary snacks and beverages is a controversial measure that has not been accepted by all school districts or schools, the decline in the presence of sugary treats has been notable.

Affordability of Health

As previously mentioned, almost every neighborhood offers fast food restaurants that are easily accessible. In the past, people have argued that healthy food is too expensive and people in poor inner-city neighborhoods cannot afford to buy it. They have argued that there is also limited access to fresh produce and organic products in these neighborhoods. So, what's the alternative for families who believe they cannot afford quality, healthy foods? You guessed it—fast food.

Mark Bittman, food journalist and author for the *New York Times*, cited the following seven reasons why people often choose fast food over home-cooked meals:

1. Fast food is cheaper.
2. There are "food desert" places in rural areas where people have to drive ten miles or more to find a supermarket.
3. People opt for fast food because they are fearful of, or challenged by, cooking.
4. Cooking seems like work.
5. Fast food is a pleasure and a crutch.
6. Hyper processed foods are convenient and virtually addictive.

7. Marketing of fast food is alluring (for example, dollar deals, family meals, and new products).

The idea that junk food is cheaper is actually a myth, though it is often thought to explain why Americans are overweight, particularly those with lower incomes. But two Big Macs, a cheeseburger, six chicken McNuggets, two medium and two small fries, and two medium and two small soda costs more than a whole chicken with vegetables, along with a simple salad and milk, which can feed a family of four. Or, you can make a few substitutions to that meal and cut the cost in half. Water can replace soda, and tasty and affordable alternatives to junk food include rice, grains, pasta, beans, fresh vegetables, canned vegetables, frozen vegetables, meat, fish, poultry, dairy products, bread, and peanut butter.

Common sense suggests that if you can drive to McDonald's you can drive to the grocery store. The bottom line is that regardless of income level, most people can afford real food. Yet people persist in wanting to find any possible reason to indulge in fast, convenient options.

Fast food restaurants and companies that prepare frozen or prepackaged foods have made it easy for people to choose unhealthy food. It certainly is faster. It seems more affordable. It's highly addictive. It's literally everywhere. Millions of dollars are spent on advertising, promotions, family meals, prizes, toys, and the latest food trends made fast. Even if the consumer opts for low-calorie, low-sodium, or fat-free foods, there are a number of chemicals and preservatives in all processed choices.

So, why do consumers still do it? Why do they choose the unhealthy over the healthy? To find the answer, another side to eating needs to be explored: emotional eating.

Chapter 9

Emotional Eating

How you react emotionally is a
choice in any situation.
— Judith Orloff

Food is more than just a way to satisfy hunger and nourish the body. Over time, food has become a means of relieving stress, influencing our emotions, and celebrating good times with others. People have learned that there are multiple ways to use food beyond meeting basic nutritional needs. In many ways, food has become connected or bound with both negative and positive emotional moments and has come to play a very different role in the everyday human experience. Food means different things to different people, and the role of food in your life has probably changed as you have grown. In early life, your parents provided food simply for nutrition. As you grew older and made food choices, you came to understand food in different ways. Food can be used as a reward – for example, a pizza party at school, ice cream for good grades, or a candy bar for good behavior. Food can be used as a punishment, such as no dessert after poor dinner behavior, being forced to finish a meal, or being made to eat unpleasant foods. Food brings people together at celebrations such as weddings and birthday parties, and is a way to self-soothe after a long day, a painful breakup, or a traumatic experience. Food can become your dear friend when people are not there for you.

Despite these powerful emotional attachments we have to food, it's important to avoid the trap of *emotional eating*, and to eat mindfully instead. But how do we actually do this? Well, first it's essential to differentiate between the desire to eat based on emotions or outside stimuli such as parents, peers, or festive occasions, and the desire to eat because of a true physical need. How can you tell the difference? According to researchers at the University of Texas Counseling and Mental Health Center, there are several differences between emotional hunger and physical hunger:

1. Emotional hunger comes on suddenly; physical hunger develops gradually.
2. When you're eating to fill a void that is not related to an empty stomach, you crave a specific food such as pizza or ice cream, and only that food will meet your need. When you eat because you're actually hungry, you are open to options.
3. Emotional hunger feels as if it needs to be satisfied instantly with the food you crave; physical hunger can wait.
4. If you're eating to satisfy an emotional need, you're more likely to keep eating even after you are full. When you're eating because you are hungry, you're more likely to stop when you are full.
5. Emotional eating can leave behind feelings of guilt; eating when you are physically hungry does not.

Stress Eating

Some people eat when they are stressed. In some ways, it's simply human nature to want to comfort and satisfy yourself to relieve the pain associated with stress. Food is an easy way to do that. Sometimes the eating occurs without thought, but sometimes it's well planned and carefully executed. Depending on your family life, the style of parenting you were exposed to, and how you learned about food, you may choose different ways to use food when you are stressed. Of course not everyone uses food in this way; people relieve stress in many ways, both healthy and unhealthy.

But if food is a stress reliever for you, it may help to take a look at your experience growing up as a way to gain insight into your own strategies associated with stress eating. If, as discussed earlier, we eat in learned ways, our childhood experiences are critical to the understanding of why we eat the way we do. How did your parents, siblings, and early peers influence your eating behaviors, and how does that affect your current eating habits?

A negative mood in response to stress has been significantly related to higher calorie consumption. In response to stress, the hormone cortisol tends to go *up*; and with consumption of excess calories it tends to go *down*. This supports the claim that there are psychophysiological influences on eating behavior. Women who are more vulnerable to mood swings as a result of added stress may be susceptible to stress-induced eating and weight gain.

In their 2009 report "Association of Eating Behaviors and Obesity with Psychosocial and Familial Influences," researchers Stephen Brown, Glenn Schiraldi, and Peggy Wrobleski made a study of eating behaviors and family influences. To determine the effect of parenting on eating behavior, they asked their study participants a series of questions about early food experiences. They used the following questions in their study, and answering the same questions might help you gain insight into how you learned about the values, roles, and impacts of food:

1. While you were growing up, did your family show love or care by offering food?
2. While growing up, how often were you offered food to comfort you when you were emotionally upset?
3. Who usually offered you this food?
4. How often did this same person eat for comfort when he or she was emotionally upset?

A 2009 study by researcher K. H. Brown on the subject of emotional eating and familial influences found that people who reported being offered food as comfort when emotionally upset as children were over 2.5 times more likely to report frequent emotional eating as young adults. Essentially, as children, these people were taught to use food as a coping skill. It makes sense that they would carry this emotional eating into young adulthood and beyond. Using food to manage emotional challenges can become a habit, which not only may trigger increased weight but also may prevent people from learning other, more effective non-food-based coping skills for easing their emotional distress.

Although emotional eating may be more common among people who struggle with weight issues, it can affect a wider group as well. People of normal weight may eat emotionally on one day, but attempt to compensate the next day by working out or dieting. Overweight emotional eaters may not be able to tap into these same kinds of coping skills. This difference in compensatory behaviors can drastically impact the future of the emotional eater.

Food as an Expression of Love

In a recent conversation concerning the human food connection, a friend of mine shared that although she does not remember her parents offering her food as a comfort during times of emotional upset, she believes that her mother-in-law often used this technique. To this day, the mother-in-law offers food as a way of showing she cares for and *loves* her family. You cannot enter her home without being offered something to eat and drink. It might be a roast that has been cooking in the crockpot all day or a frozen pizza she just bought at Sam's Club, but she will offer it regardless. She's always willing to warm something up for you or to toss a fresh salad just to feed the ones she loves. This is wonderful of her, especially after a long day of work. However, this habit of caring and loving with food may be a key reason why her husband and her children have almost always struggled with weight and overeating. My friend notices how her husband uses food in a comforting way, and she knows that some of his habits are grounded in what he learned from his mother. Once those habits are there, they are terribly hard to break or change. Although her husband realizes that there are many other kinds of rewards for successes (for example, movies, a new hat, or a new game or book), food remains a favored choice. Similarly, although he knows that food is not the only form of comfort in times of distress, it's still a favored choice at those times.

Masking Unpleasant Emotions

Oreos, Chex Muddy Buddies, potato chips, Doritos, or popcorn can seem to be your best friends. They are always there when you need them. They will not criticize, judge, or ignore you, call you fat, or say things that make you feel ashamed of yourself.

Food is a devoted friend in that sense. You can turn to it when the mood strikes, and it will not get mad at you for being fickle. You can buy as much as you want, eat as much as you want, and still get more whenever you want. You do not have to worry about food calling you back, stealing your boyfriend, or boring you with the details of its love life. It's quite possibly the perfect friend – except for the calories, fat, sodium, and sugar it brings along.

You feel sad and lonely; you eat. You feel depressed; you eat. You feel angry; you eat. You feel frustrated; you eat. Regardless of the emotion, if you are an emotional eater, when you eat you probably feel happier for a short time. In a sense, the food has masked the emotion, so you do not feel it. But that's exactly the problem with eating to mask emotions—you are quite happy for only a short period of time. The good feelings are fleeting. Then you realize how much you ate, and the terrible pendulum swings the other way. You start to feel shame. *I ate the whole thing! Why did I do that? I'm an idiot.* You almost immediately regret it, but it's too late. Shame has already set in, and you may not even have put your spoon or the bag down yet. You might even feel sick to your stomach. Clearly, eating to mask emotion isn't effective; it actually exacerbates the emotion and brings up other negative emotions in the process.

A young child who has been raised in a home that emphasizes the use of food to soothe emotions will probably not learn better coping skills. If a child is consistently appeased with a sweet treat when he or she feels sad, the experience is no longer an emotional learning situation. Instead, it's a chance to get a treat. The treat is associated with pleasure, and the underlying sadness is smoothed over. When the feeling returns—as it surely will—the child will be looking for another sweet treat for comfort. Over time, the child becomes dependent on the treat and does not learn appropriate alternative coping skills for dealing with sadness. The feeling has been pushed away, ignored, and disregarded. The same is true for any emotion that has been linked with eating and comfort.

The problems with eating to replace coping skills are obvious. Being afforded the opportunity to learn how to respond to emotions is critical in development. We can learn about emotions on paper, in books, or on television, but it's necessary to experience emotions for real understanding. Without experiencing the true effects of shame, guilt, frustration, anxiety, and other emotions, a child is unable truly to feel emotions or learn to solve the problems that produce the emotion. Learning appropriate responses to everyday emotions through play, interactions with others, and observing others is an important part of a child's development. It's vital for children both to understand emotions and to learn to cope with them in an effective and healthy way.

Celebrating Emotions

Hooray! A special event! A party! I hope the food is going to be great! We do this all the time; we celebrate successes and accomplishments with food. We have graduation parties, baby showers, anniversary dinners, birthday parties, and countless other occasions that feature food as the main attraction. Sure, the people at these events are the most important, but food is always central. What kind of birthday would it be without a birthday cake and ice cream? If you went to a party and there was no food, what would you think? A wedding is all about the cake and the dinner; that is what guests talk about (in addition to the bride's dress, of course). We expect a fancy meal, something different, something out of the ordinary, and something better than what we eat every day. We are disappointed if the food does not measure up to our expectations.

People have always come together over food. It brings people closer. It passes down traditions from one generation to the next. It's a cultural experience. Food is a commonality and a uniting factor.

The problem with using food to celebrate is that we are pairing positive emotions with high-risk dietary situations. This is a nightmare for anyone who is trying to be smart about eating. Just as food can mask negative emotions, it can also amplify positive emotions. When eating, which is already a pleasurable experience, is paired with positive emotion, the pleasure is increased, and the tendency to overeat is greater. What's worse is that over time we will require more and more of the "good stuff" to maintain the emotional high that we feel during these celebrations. Food becomes a bit like an addictive drug.

Food Addiction

Here's the vexing conundrum of our relationship with food: it can be rightfully claimed that every single human being is "addicted" to food. Like air and water, food is sustenance. If we do not eat, we die. It's a simple and stark equation. And this necessity is the source of frequent rationalization by people who eat to excess. "But I'm *starving*," the overweight youngster will howl between meals. Or the harried office worker who announces at three in the afternoon, "I simply must have a chocolate coffee and muffin from Dunkin' Donuts, or I will *die*." What hard-hearted Scrooge would deny these suffers their nourishment?

But none of us needs a TV weight-loss show exercise guru to tell us that while we all must have food to survive, too much food is not only wasteful—it's *toxic.* And as surely as any narcotic, food can become addictive.

People might believe that their eating is out of control, but most of us know that there is always control. There is always choice. It's quite possible that while the overeater's emotions are out of control, or, more likely, that some aspect of his or her life is out of control, the eating itself can still be controlled. We all have emotional meals every now and then, but for some people it's a chronic problem. Maybe food has bound so tightly with powerful emotions that it becomes a natural reaction, almost a reflex, to eat when the feeling approaches. At the same time, it's not likely that food of any sort will serve as a solution to any of the situations that cause these feelings. Rather, food might appease and satisfy by masking the emotion temporarily, but overindulging often leads to nausea, shame, guilt, and even depression. Shame can bind to many different things, and we can get so wound up with those situations, emotions, and experiences that it's exceedingly difficult to break the cycle.

If you look at your own lifestyle and eating habits, you can probably identify plenty of times when you eat emotionally rather than to satisfy actual hunger. Most of us have done that at one time or another. The best example I can think of is dessert. We may have just eaten a balanced meal with all the nutrients, vitamins, and minerals we could possibly need, but we still want dessert. Maybe we just want something sweet to cleanse the palate, maybe that cheesecake looks too good to turn down, or maybe we have learned since childhood to expect dessert after a meal. There are so many choices, too—ice cream, cake, brownies, cupcakes, pie, cookies, and more—and there are endless varieties within each of those categories. Whatever the reason, if we are not genuinely hungry for dessert, we are eating to satisfy some sort of emotion. The extra calories will, of course, put on extra fat.

Food addiction is insidious and powerful. It's when you cannot leave the restaurant without that extra dessert. It's when you proudly diet all day and then, in the secrecy of your kitchen at night, you eat an entire cake. It's when you reward yourself with ten brownies after you've walked to the mailbox and back. You know that emotional eating could actually end up killing you even as you reach for the door to the refrigerator.

Chapter 10

Family – We Eat What We Know

> If you do not pour water on your plant, what will happen? It will slowly wither and die. Our habits will also slowly wither and die away if we do not give them an opportunity to manifest. You need not fight to stop a habit. Just do not give it an opportunity to repeat itself.
>
> — Swami Satchidanada

There's no question that both individual choices and genetics play a role in the way we do many things in our lives, including eating and exercise. There is such a thing as genetic predisposition to certain illnesses and diseases. You are likely to share some of your parents' physical traits, mental aptitudes, and so on. You are also influenced by the lifestyle choices that your parents make. If your parents smoke, you might smoke. If your parents use alcohol regularly, you might come to do so as well. If your parents believe that fast food is fabulous, you will probably enjoy it too. Similarly, if your parents are social service professionals, you might learn the importance of helping others. If your parents enjoy vegetables, you probably will too. If your parents choose an active lifestyle, it would probably be more difficult to become a couch potato in their home. Our choices of behaviors, both good and bad, are influenced by the behavior of our parents.

Each family situation is unique, and each individual makes decisions within that family. I think about some families I know that have young children. They may get into a routine of eating chicken nuggets and French fries (fast food or made at home—what's the difference really?) or macaroni and cheese or hotdogs because those are child-friendly foods. So every night it becomes the same thing. These children grow up with consistency, knowing what to expect. It may not be colorful or fun or contain any variety; the meal may not even include any fruits or vegetables. But children continue to eat a limited diet of chicken, noodles, and potatoes because it tastes good and they are comfortable with it. Perhaps these children were offered a variety of foods at one time and did not eat them, so the parents have given up and have decided to go with what works in the short term. Obviously, the effect is that the child eats the same thing over and over. There's the chicken nugget cooked to oblivion in the microwave because it's easy and fast, and it ends up not tasting like chicken at all. There's yesterday's macaroni with completely artificial powdered cheese that has absolutely *no* redeeming nutritional value, and there are French fries that may be cold from yesterday and totally disgusting or overcooked and hard from being warmed in the microwave. This is not really eating. It certainly is not healthy. It's not doing the children or the parents any favors in the long run.

Of course, there are the wonderfully positive parents who from day one have trained their children with healthy choices. I was inspired when a mom I knew labeled a muffin as a cupcake and provided banana nut or blueberry as a treat for her child. What a splendid idea! I was further inspired when my seven-year-old grandson refused to eat lunch on the first day of the school year because he did not see any healthy choices in the lunch line. How many seven-year-olds would choose not to eat lunch for that reason? His mother later found out that chicken salad had been offered for lunch that day, but, by the time he got to the cafeteria, there was none left. Amazing! So, it can be done. Educating children is the key.

At some point, it's a question of what the child is exposed to, what the parent enjoys eating, and the kind of enthusiasm about variety that parents display at mealtime. If a child is exposed only to starches, white flour foods, and highly processed snacks that taste relatively good, that is probably what the child will ask for and crave. If the child is encouraged to eat what the adults are eating and sees older family members enjoying things like hummus, zucchini, salad, and blueberries, then it's likely that the child will learn to enjoy those foods too.

As a parent, I do believe the tactic of modeling food enthusiasm really works. I have seen it work. It's truly a simple idea. Start healthy eating habits early. If you're excited about something, your enthusiasm can be contagious. Young children want to model their behavior after the adults they love, even the older siblings they adore. If those people set good examples and illustrate healthy behaviors, it makes sense that children will want to try it too.

I have heard parents say, "We tried that—giving our children vegetables and fruits—but they did not eat them." To that I say, obviously, you did not wait until your child was hungry enough!

Remember this: if you offer your child a choice of healthy and nutritious foods, he or she *will not starve*. Hunger is a powerful motivator.

The first time your child said, "I want a frozen waffle instead," you probably gave in. You probably allowed your child to avoid the vegetables because you honestly do not like them either. You probably gave up because arguing or convincing your child takes too long, and you just want to enjoy your meal in peace. You might have decided that you did not want to keep wasting food, and you would just serve something you know is tried and true, like chicken fingers and fries.

But if you actually thought about it and counted the waste of shriveled up potatoes and chicken breading that you pour down the disposal each night, when all is said and done, it's much more wasteful than a few bites of broccoli, especially after you have calculated the cost of gas to go get the fast food, the packaging, the paper, the advertising for the company that makes the food, and the energy used to microwave or cook the meal. So much waste! But that is a separate issue. The point here is that parents sometimes take the easy route in feeding their children, and this does not help anyone. I know children, I know how they learn, I know what they like, and I understand the psychology behind health, motivation, and other aspects of childrearing that do work. If a parent believes something can work, then there are all kinds of possibilities. If you're excited about food, your child will be too. If you love to shop for food and cook and bake, chances are your child will too. If you encourage healthy choices, you offer healthy options, and you remain steadfast, your child will choose healthy options. I believe it. Do you?

Teenagers

A recurring theme of this book is that children model their behavior on their parents. If the parents eat healthy foods, the child will too. That much is true.

As anyone who has raised a teenager knows, an important part of growing up is the formation of the child's unique identity. When kids arrive at puberty they begin to say, "I am *me*. I am *not* my parents." This is healthy and necessary. It's also stressful for parents, as their own sweet little kids suddenly turn into six-foot Frankensteins who seem determined make life miserable for mom and dad.

The adolescent period is one of experimentation. The child who for years ate healthy foods may explore the world of junk foods. They may also play too many video games, hang out with undesirables, and try things like alcohol and sex. It happens to nearly every parent.

This is where your years of building a solid foundation will pay off. The child who is solidly grounded in good eating habits, has a rational view of alcohol, and has known only a stable and loving environment, has a much better chance of emerging into adulthood with these values intact. The teenaged forays into fast food will quickly become tiresome, and, once curiosity has been satisfied, the good health habits learned in childhood will return.

Social and Economic Pressures

Clearly, the effects of individual choice and parenting are critical in the rearing of a healthy child. Some families have an advantage because of genetics, economic fortune, availability of nutritious food, and education that allows them to make smart choices. On the flip side, there are many families that have not been supplied this kind of social capital. There are disadvantaged families that are subject to inconsistent income, low income, lack of resources, and a lack of access to places that encourage physical exercise. How can people who do not have the necessary social capital compete in a world that is becoming more and more obese? How can these socially disadvantaged people counteract the unhealthy effects of fast food, the media, and the other obstacles that they face? It becomes a challenge that affects all of us because these issues are the ones that contribute to the obesity epidemic. It becomes the responsibility of those who are advantaged and who have access to opportunities to increase their Health Intelligence to assist those who are disadvantaged to raise their healthy living quotient.

To do this we must understand what the specific issues are, how those issues play out in the general population, and how these factors contribute to the overall picture of health throughout the world.

Chapter 11

Your Relationship to the Food Groups

The purest and truest relationship is one
that will never cause you hurt or pain.
— Dr. Benji

We all have unique food experiences, and we all feel differently about various kinds of food. We have learned about fruits and vegetables from our parents and siblings. We have tried what we have tried, and we like what we like. Until we are presented with new choices and new ways of preparing foods, I imagine that we all tend to fall into a bit of a food rut. Maybe we rely on the old favorites that are easy to prepare, easy to find in the store, and taste good to us. I love tomatoes, corn, and beans; those are my go-to vegetables.

As adults, we may learn to branch out into new directions with food. Maybe our new friends have encouraged us to try sushi or crab legs or Brussels sprouts prepared with Parmesan cheese. Maybe a spouse has introduced us to kale salad or spaghetti squash or something else we had not tried before, or maybe food trends have affected what we taste as adults. There's a new vegetarian restaurant, food truck, or whole foods store that just opened up that we'd like to try. Whatever the case, our food experiences continue to grow. We do not have to remain stuck eating what we learned to enjoy as children. We can expand our horizons and try new things that we might actually enjoy as adults. If we do not open our minds to all the possibilities, we will be missing out on some really tasty foods.

My friend Gloria says that she never liked gyros until she was about twenty-five years old. She had never tasted a crab leg until she was in her late twenties and only recently came to enjoy kale. She asks herself, "Where have I been? And why did I not try these things before?" She thinks she was a finicky eater as a child. She liked chicken fingers, French fries, macaroni and cheese, and a few fruits and vegetables. She states that her parents encouraged her to try all kinds of foods, but she had no interest in exploring new things. It was not until she had friends, money, and access to new places that she decided to branch out and try new foods. She is now exceedingly glad she has that opportunity. Foods she now enjoys are most kinds of fish, sushi, oranges, cauliflower, and Brussels sprouts. She likes to be adventurous and creative with food, so she is always willing to try something new. She is often amazed at her new creations.

One of the best ways to take inventory of your eating habits is to look at each food category and put your ideas on to paper. This way, you can look at your habits with perspective and return to the paper for reference as you begin a new food adventure.

The Vegetables Survey

Starting with vegetables, think about the choices you have made in the past, what you like, what you do not like, what you have not tried, what you would like to try, and other thoughts you have about vegetables. Think about your childhood experiences.

Were you forced to eat vegetables? Did you hate the whole idea of green leafy textures? Was mealtime uncomfortable for you in some way, so you associate vegetables with anxiety? Really reflect on your eating and begin to be mindful about where you have been and how it has brought you to the point you are now.

Take a few minutes to inventory your relationship with vegetables. For each vegetable, place a check mark in every column that is relevant.

Not only will it help you identify what you like and what you do not like, but also it might encourage you to try something new so you can continue to expand the variety of foods in your repertoire.

When you're finished, take a look at your vegetable inventory. What do you notice? What stands out for you? Are you interested to see how many vegetables you like or do not like, or have never even heard of?

VEGETABLE	I have tried…	I love…	I like…	I don't like…	I've never heard of…	I plan to try…
Acorn squash						
Alfalfa sprouts						
Artichoke						
Arugula						
Asparagus						
Avocado (fruit)						
Adzuki beans						
Banana squash						
Bean sprouts						
Beet						
Black beans						
Black-eyed peas						
Bok choy						
Borlotti beans						
Breadfruit						
Broad beans						
Broccoflower						
Broccoli						
Brussels sprouts						
Butternut squash						
Cabbage						
Calabrese						
Carrot						
Cauliflower						
Cayenne pepper						
Celeriac						
Celery						
Chard						
Chickpeas or Garbanzo beans						

Chili pepper						
Chives						
Collard greens						
Corn						
Corn salad						
Cucumber						
Daikon						
Eggplant (fruit)						
Endive						
Fiddleheads						
Frisee						
Garlic						
Gem squash						
Ginger						
Green						
Green beans						
Habanera						
Horseradish						
Hubbard squash						
Jalapeno						
Jerusalem artichoke						
Jicama						
Kale						
Kidney beans						
Kohlrabi						
Leek						
Lentils						
Lettuce						
Lima beans or Butter beans						
Mung beans						
Mushrooms						
Mustard greens						

Navy beans						
Nettles						
New Zealand spinach						
Okra						
Onion						
Orange pepper						
Paprika						
Parsley						
Parsnip						
Patty pans						
Peas						
Pinto beans Runner beans						
Potato						
Pumpkin						
Purple pepper						
Radicchio						
Radish						
Red pepper						
Rhubarb						
Rutabaga						
Rutabaga						
Salsify						
Shallot						
Skirret						
Snap peas						
Soy beans						
Spaghetti squash						
Spinach						
Spring onion, green onion or scallion						
Sunchoke						

Sweet potato						
Tabasco pepper						
Taro						
Tat soi						
Tomato (fruit)						
Turnip						
Wasabi						
Water chestnut						
Watercress						
White radish						
Yam						
Yellow pepper						
Zucchini						

Vegetables I like...

Once you have inventoried your vegetables, get to know them in a new way. Start with your positive experiences first and choose a vegetable that you selected as one that you love.

Take a few minutes to answer the following questions about the vegetables you love and the ones you dislike; both reflections can help inform and might change the way you think about vegetables:

1. What do you love about that vegetable?
2. Can you think of a happy or positive memory from childhood that you associate with that food?
3. List a few words you associate with that vegetable.
4. What is your favorite way to prepare this vegetable?
5. What else do you usually serve with this vegetable?
6. With whom do you often share this vegetable?
7. Of what season, event, holiday, or special occasion does this vegetable remind you?

I dislike...

Now, think about some of the vegetables you *dislike* in the inventory. This is where you will want to dig a bit deeper into your childhood experiences and find out more about why you do not enjoy those vegetables.

Feel free to journal about the answers if you honestly want to get to know more about your vegetables and experiences. Of course, you do not have to do this all at once; that would be overwhelming and time-consuming. Just pick a few vegetables to begin with.

Ask yourself the following questions and really answer them:

1. Pick one of the foods you listed as a "don't like."

2. Why don't you like that vegetable?
3. What is your memory of the food the first time you tried it and the memory that comes to mind when you imagine the vegetable?
4. How was it prepared when you ate it?
5. Where were you when you ate it?
6. Who was with you?
7. What are some ways this vegetable could be prepared?
8. How could you pair that food with other foods that you like (for example, can you top it with cheese, a little butter, or sour cream, cook it with bacon, or add garlic)?

Continue this exercise with each vegetable you have identified as a "do not like." Then, explore new recipes online to find out how you might prepare that vegetable in a new way. You might learn something, and you might grow to like a vegetable you once disliked or even hate now, or you might still dislike it. The nice part about trying vegetables is that there are so many from which you can choose. You are bound to find some new ones to add to your weekly menu.

I'd like to try....

Now make a list of a few of the foods you would like to try. Do a little research on recipes that feature that vegetable. When you shop, make a conscious effort to purchase a new vegetable and try out the new recipe; just one new vegetable each time you shop is an easy way to begin. Be sure to taste the vegetable raw, take a minute to smell of the vegetable, and get to know a little bit about it before you prepare it. It's completely okay if you do not like a new vegetable right away. Try it again later prepared in a new way.

Vegetables I've never heard of…

Choose one of the vegetables you have never heard of and do a little internet research to find out what it is. Just Google it and learn a few facts. Get to know the nutritional value of the food, how it can help your body, and a few ways to prepare it. Add it to your shopping list and test out one of the recipes. Make the integration of the new food easy. Think about adding the new vegetable to a salad or soup. Be sure to focus on seasonal vegetables and local vegetables for the best, natural flavors.

Your Feelings About Fruit

Look at the fruit statements below. Check if they are true or not true about you.

TRUE or NOT TRUE:

______ I eat five servings of fruit every day.

______ I eat some fruit, but not five servings each day.

______ I don't eat much fruit.

______ I dislike most kinds of fruit.

______ I buy fruit, but I never seem to eat it; it goes bad too fast.

______ I eat fruit, but not much variety, mostly apples, oranges, and bananas.

______ Fruit is too expensive; I can't afford it!

______ Cutting fruit, taking out pits, and removing seeds is too much work.

______ I love fruit juices, fruit popsicles, fruit cups, and canned fruit.

______ I prefer fresh fruit to prepackaged fruit.

______ Fruit makes a great snack.

______ I eat lots of fruit in the summer, but it's hard to do that in the winter.

______ I like to experiment with different fruit dishes, smoothies, and desserts.

Just as you did with the vegetable inventory, take a look at the fruits in the chart below and how you feel about them. For each fruit, place a check mark in each column that is relevant.

FRUITS	I have tried…	I plan to try…	I like…	I eat frequently
Apple				
Apricot				
Banana				
Bilberry				
Blackberry				
Blackcurrant				
Blueberry				
Breadfruit				
Cantaloupe				
Cherimoya				
Cherry				
Clementine				
Currant				
Damson				
Date				
Dragon fruit				
Durian				
Elderberry				
Feijoa				
Gooseberry				
Grape				
Grapefruit				
Guava				
Honeydew melon				
Huckleberry				
Jackfruit				
Jambul				
Kiwi fruit				
Kumquat				
Lemon				
Lime				

Lychee				
Mandarine				
Mango				
Musk Melon				
Nectarine				
Orange				
Peach				
Pear				
Physalis				
Pineapple				
Pitaya				
Plum/prune				
Pomegranate				
Pomelo				
Purple Mangosteen				
Raisin				
Rambutan				
Raspberry				
Redcurrant				
Rock melon				
Salai berry				
Satsuma				
Star fruit				
Strawberry				
Tangerine				
Ugli fruit				
Watermelon				
Western raspberry				
Ziziphus Mauritania				

You probably eat more fruit than you think

Did you know that one serving of fruit is only ½ cup of grapes or one small apple? Some people do not realize how many servings of fruits and vegetables they are actually getting in a day. Everything is supersized, so, if you are eating fruits and vegetables, you might actually be getting pretty close to your daily recommended five to nine servings.

The Mayo Clinic offers online readers some useful fruit quantities that equal one serving. Use this easy list to make sure you get the right amount of fruit each day:

4 apricots
1 extra small banana
¾ cup of blackberries
¾ cup of blueberries
¾ cup of cubed pineapple
1 cup of cubed cantaloupe, honeydew melon, or papaya
½ cup of cubed mango
12 cherries
3 dates
½ of a grapefruit
½ of a pear
17 small grapes
1 kiwi
1 small nectarine
1 small orange
1 medium peach
2 small plums
2 small tangerines
1 cup of raspberries

1 ¼ cup of strawberries
1 ¼ cup of cubed watermelon
1/3 to ½ cup of real fruit juice

You can find additional information about dried fruit servings and specifics on fruit juices at http://www.mayoclinic.com/health/diabetes-diet/DA00070. With this information, it's easy to track how much fruit you are eating.

Just think, if you make a fruit smoothie and drink your fresh fruit, you've got several servings in one glass! Or, try new ways to eat your fruit—for example, smoothies, popsicles, pie, cereal toppings, with milk, in a salad, with chocolate, on fruit skewers, and yogurt dip.

Your Relationship With Protein

We used to call this category of foods the "meat group," but, with revisions to the food pyramid and the increase in people who are choosing vegetarian lifestyles and other alternatives that do not include meat, it is now called the "protein group." The protein category contains a variety of foods, including meat, seafood, shellfish, eggs, beans, peas, nuts, and seeds. These foods are high in protein (10 grams or higher) and should include low fat selections.

With this expanded view of protein, consider your relationship to the various categories by answering the following questions:

1. Do you eat meat? ________If yes, how often? __________
2. What kind of meat? ______white meat only _______red meat only________ both
3. Do you choose lean meats (for example, 90/10)? ________
4. Do you have any specific philosophical/ethical/religious

beliefs that impact what kinds of meats and proteins you choose? (Describe them here. ______________________

5. What kinds of meat do you prefer? (Check all that apply)
   Pork ______
   Chicken ______
   Beef ______
   Turkey ______
   Lamb ______
   Veal ______
   Other (duck, venison) ______
6. I get most of my protein from:
   Meat ______
   Seafood ______
   Eggs ______
   Beans and Peas ______
   Nuts and Seeds ______
   Other ______
7. When I was a child, most of my protein came from: ____
   ____
8. What does the phrase "meat and potatoes" mean to you and your family?
   ____
9. Do you like seafood and shellfish? ________________
10. How often do you eat it? ________________
11. Do you prepare it at home? ________________
12. How often do you eat eggs? ________________
13. What's your favorite way to eat eggs and why? __________
    ____

14. How often do you include beans and peas in your meals?

    ____

15. What kinds of beans and peas are your favorites?

    ____

Did you know that only one quarter of your plate should be protein? This could be an egg, ¼ cup of beans, or one ounce of meat.

The USDA suggests a wide variety of proteins and lean or low fat choices. If you're a big meat eater, try going meatless one night per week to begin. Then, challenge yourself to go a week without eating meat. If you cut meat out of your diet, you'll be eating healthier and will cut down on certain fats that your body does not need. Replace meat with other proteins and see how you feel!

Your Feelings About Grains

The grain category (formerly the bread group) is also an important part of a healthy diet. The grain category includes barley, buckwheat, bulgur, corn, emmo, grano, kamut grain, kañiwa, millet, oats, quinoa, rice, rye, sorghum, spelt, teff, triticale, wheat, and wild rice. Now, if you're like me, you have probably never heard of some of those grains and you probably stick to the common ones like wheat, rice, corn, and oats.

For more information on the other not-so-popular but incredibly healthy grains, how to find them, and how to use them, and nutritional information, visit the Whole Grain Council website at http://www.wholegrainscouncil.org/whole-grains-101/whole-grains-a-to-z/.

The Whole Grain Council website provides information to the

public about the different types of whole grains, nutritional benefits, dietary suggestions, factual information, recipes, news, and more.

The USDA suggests that people consume three to five servings of grains per day.

Here is what one serving looks like:

1/2 cup cooked brown rice (or other cooked grain).

1/2 cup cooked 100% whole grain pasta.

1/2 cup cooked hot cereal such as oatmeal.

1 ounce uncooked whole grain pasta, brown rice, or other grain.

1 slice 100% whole grain bread.

1 very small (1 oz.) 100% whole grain muffin.

1 cup 100% whole grain ready-to-eat cereal.

There is a tremendous push toward whole grains with all kinds of products, including bread, pastries, cereals, and crackers. The emphasis is on reducing bleached, white flour, processed foods and replacing them with whole grains. There are many companies that offer whole grain breakfast products; for example, General Mills has introduced the following whole grain cereals for adults and kids:

http://www.wholegrainnation.eatbetteramerica.com

General Mills cereals have between eight and sixteen grams of whole grain per serving, which can help you to reach the recommended daily amount of 48 grams quickly. Having a nutritious breakfast is a terrific start to your day, and breakfast with whole grains offers numerous benefits such as promoting heart health, minimizing the risk of cancer, lowering the effects of diabetes, keeping your digestion regular, and helping to manage your weight. Most food packaging has clear labels that help to identify products with whole grains; General Mills suggests that consumers look for the large white check as an indication that the product is made with whole grain (http://wholegrainnation.eatbetteramerica.com/).

Now take the time to get to know your grain-eating habits. Answer the questions below to gain some insight into your experience with grains and whole grains.

Did your parents purchase wheat or white bread? __________

Did your parents trim the crust off your peanut butter and jelly sandwiches when you were little? __________________________

What kind of bread do you purchase now as an adult? Is it whole grain? ____

Do you eat a variety of grains or do you eat the same kind routinely? ____

Which grains are contained in your favorite cereals? Is the grain listed as the first ingredient? ______________________________

When you purchase crackers or chips, which grain do you usually choose? _______________________________________

When you go to the grocery store, there are so many choices that sometimes it's difficult to determine what's healthy, what has whole grain, and what snacks to avoid. Luckily, many companies have large print on their packaging to identify whole grains. But the savvy consumer must look further than that to determine calorie count, fat content, sodium, sugar, and so on.

While whole grains are a signal that the product has some nutrients you need, you still need to read the entire label to know what you're getting. In addition to the information on packaging, other sources including magazines, articles, books, and newspapers are available to offer lots of advice on what you should choose for nutritional reasons. You still have to read the fine print to get all the details, and you still have to try the food to see if you like the taste.

If nothing else, there are plenty of resources to help you narrow down your search for the best of the best. Even the most health savvy among us can scarcely determine what is best by looking at a single package.

Your Feelings About Dairy Products

Everyone has a different relationship with dairy products. Some people grew up drinking milk and eating ice cream for dessert. Others hate the idea of cottage cheese and get an upset stomach at the thought of drinking a glass of milk. I love dairy products. I grew up drinking milk every morning and still try to drink a glass of milk every day. I have now grown a bit lactose intolerant, so I have replaced the traditional 2% milk with unsweetened almond milk. I love butter, but I do not use it excessively. I indulge in a few scoops of Haagen-Dazs rum raisin ice cream every now and then, and some cottage cheese, low fat yogurt, and a little cheese provide me with the balance I need from the dairy group.

What's your relationship with dairy products? Take a little time to reflect on your experiences with foods such as ice cream, milk, cottage cheese, yogurt, cheese, cream, sour cream, cream cheese, and butter.

Check the following statements that apply to you:

I'm allergic to dairy products. ______

I have strong negative reactions to dairy products. ______

I cannot stop eating ice cream. ______

I love cheese on everything, every kind of cheese and extra cheese too. ______

I drink a glass of milk every day. ______

I almost always choose low-fat dairy products. ______

I rarely eat dairy products. ______

Dairy products are too fattening. ______

Low-fat dairy products do not taste good to me. ______

I choose soy or rice-based products in place of milk-processed foods. ______

According to the 2005 Dietary Guidelines published by the National Dairy Council, children do not get enough of essential nutrients such as calcium, potassium, and magnesium, which are found in high quantities in dairy products. Dairy foods are a good source of nine essential nutrients: calcium, potassium, phosphorus, protein, riboflavin, niacin, and Vitamins A, D, and B12. Studies showed that increasing a child's intake of nutrient-rich dairy foods (for example, milk, cheese, and yogurt) improves the quality of his or her diet. Scientific findings also show that the recommended daily serving of dairy food does not affect a child's body fat levels in negative ways and may actually protect against adding excess body fat.

According to the United States Department of Agriculture (USDA), the following items each equal one serving of dairy:

1 cup of milk

1/1 pint container of milk

½ cup of evaporated milk

1 container of yogurt

1 cup of yogurt

½ cup of shredded cheese

2 slices of processed cheese

½ cup of ricotta cheese

2 cups of cottage cheese

1 cup of pudding made with milk

1 cup of frozen yogurt

1 cup of calcium-fortified soy milk

1 ½ cups of ice cream

This is an interesting list of foods and quantities because, when you look at it, you might think, "Great, I can eat one and a half cups of ice cream!" But don't forget that when you read the label of a gallon of ice cream, the recommended serving is often one-half to one cup. One and a half cups of ice cream will give you the recommended daily allowance of dairy nutrients, but remember you're also getting calories, fat, and sugars in that serving too. As your Health Intelligence quotient increases you'll become increasingly aware that some products are full of essential vitamins and nutrients, but that there are also negatives to look out for.

We've covered a wealth of information about healthy foods and your own personal eating habits. This is just one piece of the puzzle when it comes to having Health Intelligence. You may want to take your own reflective journey about the other facets of Health Intelligence as well. You may want to assess where you are with your environmental awareness; your spiritual past, present, and future; your physical activity regimen; and your relationships. Some basic questions about these areas are included in the Health Intelligence questionnaire at http//www.drbenji.com. Please take time to evaluate how you can improve your understanding of where you have been, where you are right now, and where you want to go with your overall health.

Chapter 12

Efforts to Improve Health Intelligence

When we least expect it, life sets us a challenge to test our courage and willingness to change; at such a moment, there is no point in pretending that nothing has happened or in saying that we are not yet ready. The challenge will not wait. Life does not look back. A week is more than enough time for us to decide whether or not to accept our destiny.
— Paulo Coelho

Only a revolution in consciousness will save children from obesity. We have to change the old ways of thinking about food and the total health of our bodies. Such a change requires a paradigm shift.

Such shifts can happen. For example, as recently as World War One many more military personnel died from infections and communicable diseases than from severe wounds on the battlefield. It was only after better medical treatments were developed and used that the soldiers stopped dying from disease and less traumatic injuries. There was a change in how the illnesses were handled. Something was wrong, so doctors and researchers set out to find a solution. The old way of thinking about addressing that crisis had to change because it was not working. A paradigm shift occurred. This type of shift can only happen, however, when the problem becomes important enough to both to those who the problem most greatly impacts and those in a position to act.

Parents and educators alike must now take a stand to change the direction of unhealthy habits among the young. The old way of thinking has caused a tremendous strain on the health care system and an escalation of a variety of diseases. Because thirty to fifty percent of calories that children eat on a daily basis come from their meals at school, a change in food choices served in U.S. school cafeterias will make an enormous impact. The "aha-aha" moment is now. Enough light has been shed on the obesity problem that we know we have to change our approach to feeding our young if we do not want their life spans to be shortened.

Educators have to make curriculum changes to educate children on the importance of healthy eating. Today, learning about appropriate basic health practices is just as critical as learning reading, writing, and arithmetic. Children will need to be involved in interactive hands-on approaches to nutrition in order to feel in a direct way what it means to be healthy. This direct experience is necessary in order for change to occur. The ancient Chinese proverb says it best: "If you give a man a fish, you feed him for a day. If you teach a man to fish, you feed him for a lifetime." In order to make lasting change, it's always best to help individuals learn the skill that will allow them to function independently to allow for a lifetime of wellness. Schools must therefore seek "buy-in" from all stakeholders within the school community to be able to meet this difficult challenge.

Michelle Obama, the First Lady of the United States, has started a remarkable trend. She has inspired the nation by doing the following:

- ✓ Starting a national conversation.
- ✓ Planting a vegetable garden at the White House.
- ✓ Exploring and connecting with children to find their interest in nutrition.
- ✓ Getting children engaged in planting, nurturing, harvesting and writing about vegetables in a relatable and friendly manner.
- ✓ Getting commitments from school districts, mayors, governors, television networks, pediatricians, and sports teams.
- ✓ Getting funding through the legislature to aid in implementing and providing the necessary resources needed to encourage change.

Mrs. Obama has gone to meet with individuals from various organizations to communicate the importance of saving the lives of children. Mrs. Obama articulates that she is willing to move heaven and earth to do the best for her own two children, and she believes that all parents have the will to do the same for their children. Some need more support than others, but, as a nation, we can provide this support. So, what has been done so far?

Positive Messages on Television, the Media, and in the Public Sphere

Researchers have found several ways that television viewing affects the rise in childhood obesity. As a result, efforts have been made to limit unhealthy advertising aimed at young children and to emphasize positive, healthy, active lifestyles in programming and advertisements. These efforts are an excellent beginning to an ongoing task of informing the public about health and nutrition, despite the advertising that continues to emphasize the unhealthy. This kind of advertising is not going away; we just have to learn how to combat it effectively.

Here are some healthy initiatives for the whole family:

Verb campaign

It is what you *do*. The mission is to increase and maintain physical activity among tweens (ages nine to thirteen). The goals are to:

- Increase knowledge and improve attitudes and beliefs about tweens' regular participation in physical activity.
- Increase parental and influencer support and encouragement of tweens' participation in physical activity.
- Heighten awareness of options and opportunities for tween participation in physical activity.
- Facilitate opportunities for tweens to participate in regular physical activity.
- Increase and maintain the number of tweens who regularly participate in physical activity.

Five a Day for Better Health Program

This initiative encourages people of all ages to consume five to nine fruits and vegetables every day for better health.

Let's Just Play!

This program is an effort to get kids moving, to get kids away from television, and to promote an active lifestyle. Nickelodeon's website features one hundred ways to play, tip sheets, clips, a tracker to keep progress, and lots of activities to get children motivated and active.

Play 60!

Play 60! Is a national youth health and fitness campaign focused on increasing the wellness of young fans by encouraging them to be active for at least sixty minutes a day.

Elmocize!

Elmocize became popular in 1996 and was designed to get kids moving with their favorite furry red monster. Health has always been included in Sesame Workshop's curriculum, but since 2004 it has been integrating messages about healthy eating into its daily shows.

In 2006, Sesame Workshop initiated a multimedia outreach program; they sent kits filled with health information to child care providers. In 2012, Mrs. Obama made an appearance to foster healthy habits for life.

Boobah

Boobah encourages children to move, dance, and create stories.

Georgia Shape

Georgia's governor, Nathan Deal, has spearheaded the Georgia Shape Initiative for children. He has formed a network of partners, agencies, and athletic teams including the Atlanta Falcons, the Atlanta Braves, the Georgia Department of Public Health, and the Georgia Department of Education. These partners have committed to improving the health of our young people by offering assistance and opportunity to achieve a greater level of overall fitness.

Health Corps

This organization was founded by Dr. Oz and his wife, Lisa, to find ways that will combat childhood obesity. They are focused on providing support and awareness in schools throughout this nation.

The media can provide knowledge about healthy habits and access to this knowledge, but this still might not change behavior. While the media can increase awareness of health-related issues, there is less evidence that the media can stimulate behavior change. People seem to love their junk food and kids who are exposed to it early cannot seem to get enough.

Political Efforts

President Obama and the First Lady have made it clear that health and nutrition are a main concern, and they have made efforts to improve the status of children's health in the United States. In 2010, President Obama and Congress focused on improving children's health by enacting the Healthy, Hunger-Free Kids Act. This act was designed to increase funding to improve school meals, to modify nutrition standards for all foods served in schools, and to provide better guidelines about food safety in schools.

In 2012, President Obama identified childhood obesity and nutrition as key initiatives. He revisited the Childhood Nutrition Act and asked schools to remove cakes, candies, sugary and salty snacks, and soda pop from school vending machines. Simultaneously, there was a push to encourage children to eat more whole grains, fruits, and vegetables.

The president also intends to increase the number of students who receive school breakfast and lunch, and hopes to connect local farmers with schools in order to provide more parent and child education on the subject of nutrition. The results of these initiatives remain to be seen.

In addition to attempts to limit sweets, some companies have decided to counteract unhealthiness altogether by removing existing vending machines and replacing them with healthy vending options. A company called Vendu-cation allows schools to fill their own vending machines with healthy choices that students will purchase.

Other companies such as Healthy You Vending and Sprout Healthy Vending are marketing vending machines to entrepreneurs who believe in the political push toward better health and want to provide healthy vending options to students. Apparently, this effort is just as successful as previous vending alternatives; it's already a $40+ billion business and is steadily growing each year.

Prevention

It's clear that many companies and individuals have made healthy eating a priority. The media have responded with positive viewing choices and positive health messages. Political efforts continue to improve the offerings of food in public schools. But efforts should not stop there. Rather than focusing on how to combat the messages and problems that are already out there, we must also focus on preventative measures.

Prevention should be a primary goal in reducing childhood and adult obesity. We will have the greatest chance to successfully reverse the obesity epidemic if we take three steps: 1) recognize it as a crisis, 2) make it a funded government and public health priority, and 3) bring stakeholders together to mount an effective public health campaign in the prevention and early treatment of obesity.

From infancy, prevention should include the encouragement of healthy eating and healthy living. Prevention should have a whole-person approach that addresses sleeping habits, dental care, relationships, mental health, and overall physical health, as well as healthy eating. Prevention should include education, information, and opportunities for action. Building Health Intelligence is a lifelong process that has to begin early in life, and involves commitment and consistency. With this type of investment from individuals who are dedicated to improve, change is possible.

Activating Prior Knowledge—Learning From What We Already Know

In 1992, the U.S. Department of Agriculture came up with a graphic to represent healthy eating and the different food groups. The Food

Pyramid was designed to give consumers an easy way to access information about serving sizes or the recommended daily portions of different food categories with a visual reminder. This pyramid suggests eating the most from the grain group followed by fruits and vegetables and, then, the other food groups.

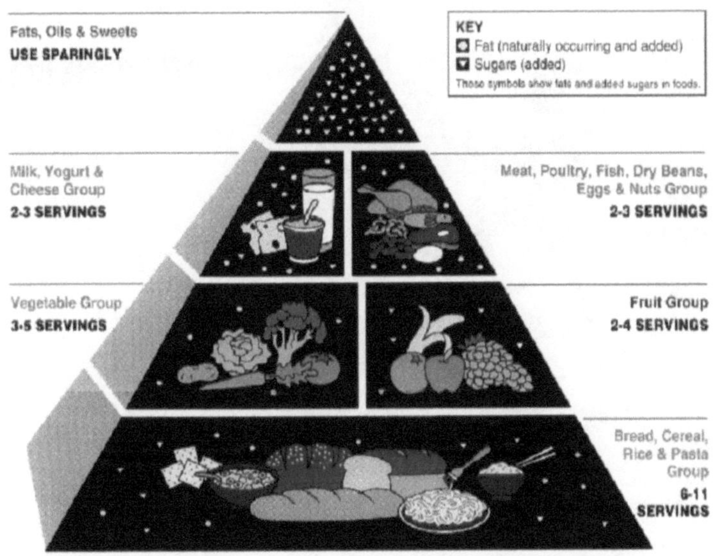

Food Portion Pyramid

Over time, the food pyramid has been altered to incorporate new information about food trends. In 2005, the USDA released a revised food pyramid that focused on the newest dietary guidelines developed by the USDA and the Department of Health and Human Services. The guidelines are updated every five years.

The following pyramid, designed by the USDA in 2005, shows a larger emphasis on fruits and vegetables, attention to beans as an important part of the protein group, and a diminished emphasis on sugars, fats, and oils. Additionally, the figure on the stairs is a graphic reminder of the importance of physical activity. This was an attempt by the USDA to encourage consumers to add physical activity into the daily routine in addition to healthy eating. The USDA recommends thirty minutes of exercise per day for adults and sixty minutes of exercise per day for children and teens.

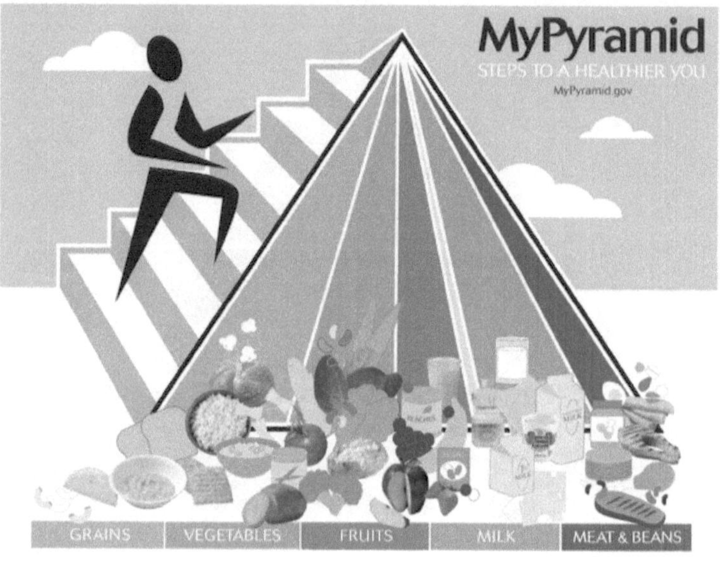

While the pyramid idea was effective, in 2011 the USDA decided to make its content more readily applicable to eating and what the portions might actually look like on a common visual—the plate. The graphic was changed to a plate that displayed the five food groups for healthy eating and quantity comparisons. This makes it easy to make sure you are getting the right mix of foods. The USDA suggests that, before you eat, you think about what goes on your plate.

The plate shows that the groups are more equal in value and

portion size. In addition, the fat, sugar, and oil group has essentially been eliminated from the picture. This suggests that fats, sugars, and oils should be eaten in small amounts and should not to be included in regular meals

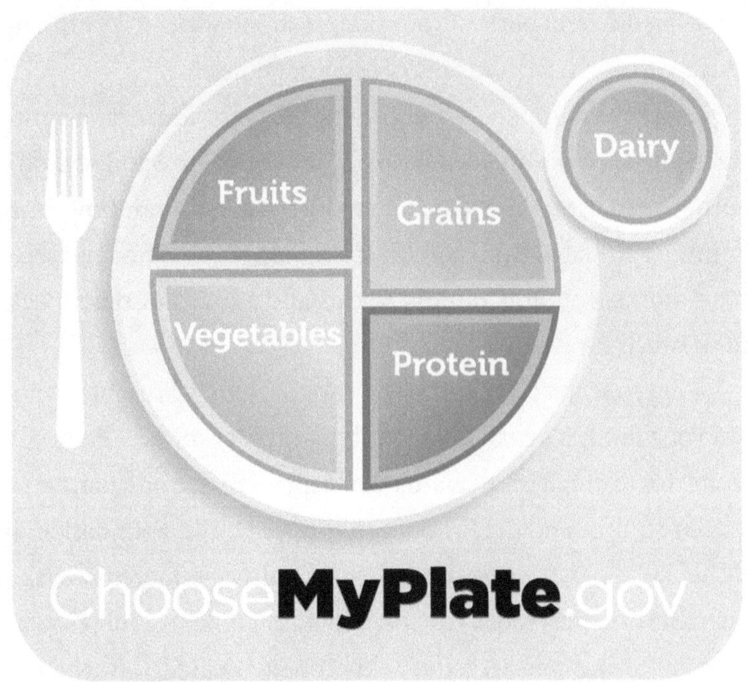

http://www.choosemyplate.gov/

Another program that tries to make healthy eating a painless process, especially for children, is the 5 A Day for Better Health Program. A U.S. nutrition campaign to encourage children to eat more fruits and vegetables, the 5 A Day for Better Health Program was started in 1991 and is a public-private partnership of the National Cancer Institute, the Produce for Better Health Foundation, the USDA, Centers for Disease Control, the American Cancer Society, and other national health organizations. Getting kids to focus on this program is an easy way to encourage healthy eating. Additionally, eating "five a day the color way" helps to encourage children to choose colorful fruits and vegetables, including a variety of reds, oranges, greens, purples, whites, and yellows. Each color group is responsible for healing different parts of your body; eating a wide variety can help to ensure that you get a variety of essential nutrients.

Numerous companies, publishers, bloggers, and organizations have capitalized on the idea of five a day the color way. Do a quick Internet search on "5 a day," "eat your colors," "rainbow in my tummy," and related word combinations and you will find numerous books, worksheets and games for kids and adults, lessons, articles, and so much more.

Eating your colors is a fun way to look at getting the right nutrition from your food; it's easy to remember and easy to do. The original website that featured the five-a-day concept was based on a partnership between Sunkist and the Produce for Better Health Foundation; the website, 5aday.org, has now become fruitsandveggiesmorematters.org, which features, tips, tools, recipes, and lots of other useful resources. There are also many websites with content geared toward young children. You can find games, activities, coloring pages, recipes, and other fun ways to encourage healthy eating.

(http://www.foodchamps.org)

After a little review of the basics—the food groups and how they have changed over time—you have the foundation necessary for moving forward with healthy eating.

One of the most powerful strategies in maintaining a healthy eating routine is knowing how to read the nutrition labels on food packages. The information can seem overwhelming and difficult to understand at first, but with a few easy tips you can have a better idea about exactly what you're getting in a product.

Each food label in the United States is set up in the same way with categories defined in the same place each time so that, once you learn the tips, you'll always be able to find the nutritional information you're looking for. You can review the label while you are in the grocery store and comparison shop across brands or products. You can compare sodium counts, fiber grams, vitamins, calories, or whatever details you want to compare for your diet. If the label lists natural ingredients first, then, it means fewer sweeteners and less sugar has been added. By the same token, if the label ingredient list is short, it's probably much closer to the real, authentic thing than if the label reads like a short story with words you cannot pronounce. Also, you should look for low saturated fat and compare the full fat and fat-free options.

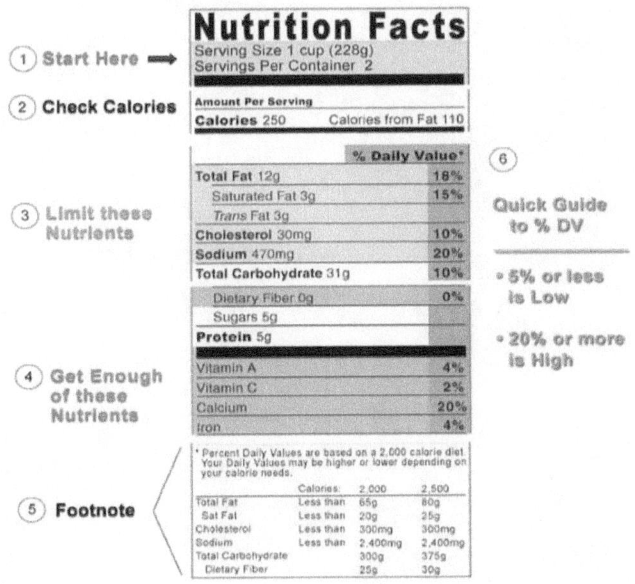

(http://www.foodpyramid.com/nutrition-facts-label)

Additionally, before you use the product, it's necessary to look at the label again to make sure you're serving the correct portion size. Portions that are too large can easily contribute to extra calories, extra fat, and extra weight gain. Read the labels. Reread the labels.

Chapter 13

Healthy Eating 101

Health and intellect are the two blessings of life.
— Menander

In the twenty-first century, healthy eating continues to be a serious challenge for American society. We know that we should eat fruits, vegetables, grains, and proteins. We know that we should eat in moderation, taking appropriate portion sizes and smaller meals. We know that we should avoid processed foods, fast foods, fat, and sugars wherever possible. But why don't we do it? Do we make choices out of laziness, convenience, affordability, or simply because we have become used to making poor eating choices?

Certainly, healthy options are available to us wherever we live and however much we have to spend on food, but the processed foods seem to be too inviting to resist. In some cases we have developed a craving for those foods. Unhealthy food has become an addiction that is extremely hard to break. After all, we are constantly exposed to messages about food in the form of digital media, in print, at restaurants, at fast food restaurants, and on television. Cooking shows such as *Cupcake Wars, Cake Boss, Chopped, The Best Thing I Ever Ate,* and *Next Food Show Star* are all about food. How can we make the biggest bakery monstrosity? How can we combine ingredients in a way that have never been done before? How can we outdo the newest fat-saturated burger, pizza, or donut? How do we take on the deepest-rooted and unhealthiest food addictions when advertisements luring people to try to these foods are part of the fabric of our culture?

Don't get me wrong—I love food. I love a succulent turkey burger with onions and mushrooms and, once in a while, with a little cheese. I love a delicious meat and vegetable pizza. As much as the next girl I love a healthy serving of apple pie à la mode, not to mention a generous serving of rich bread pudding with some vanilla ice cream. I love food shows. Mostly I watch for inspiration, for the awe of food, for gustatory satisfaction, and for the newest and healthiest recipes. I relish the creativity that people have with food, pushing the limits of what's possible and what can be mixed together to form the next sensational food invention. There is something fascinating about food. We eat it every day, there are a million varieties, and it seems like there are never-ending possibilities of dishes to create. Food is excellent. Food is delicious. Food is an expression of creativity.

Hmm . . . That makes sense. Creativity goes hand-in-hand with food preparation and, therefore, eating choices. So, does it also make sense that people who have not fully tapped into their creativity may not make healthy food choices? Or does it just mean that they have not yet opened their minds to all the possibilities of food enjoyment? I see food as a way to engage my creativity—a challenge—but if someone else sees food purely as a way to affect a change in their emotional well being, then perhaps that person does not engage as readily with the healthy qualities of food.

I enjoy food. I choose to improve my Health Intelligence. I have an interest in this area and want to develop it. So I read, I listen, I watch, I observe, and I learn. I understand what is valuable about food and what makes it taste good; those two concepts create the perfect blend for any dish. I believe that food does not have to be nasty tasting to be healthy for you. Then again, I am a lover of Lima beans and spaghetti squash, which is not typical of eat-to-survive foodies. Maybe it's because I grew up in a household where I had two parents who enforced family dinners together every afternoon. It's that practice that I extended to my children. We ate together whenever we could. Everyone participated in mealtime, whether it was preparation of the food, setting the table, clearing the table, or doing dishes. Dinnertime was a family event in which everyone had a role. There was dialogue about the day, a sharing of information, a plan for the rest of the evening, and a plan to complete homework. Sometimes dinner would be spaghetti and meatballs with a salad. At other times it was chicken, green beans, mashed potatoes and salad. Maybe it was fish, which was not a favorite for the girls, Brussels sprouts, or liver and cabbage that had to be forced down. But whatever the dish was, it was eaten together.

Eating was a positive experience for my family. It was pleasurable. My children were encouraged to try whatever was being served, and to finish what was on their plates, but I never punished or rewarded them with food. We had snacks and dessert too, but as a parent I was careful to avoid the most sugary cereals and soda pop. Processed snacks and desserts were never in abundance. We did not eat much fast food. I enjoyed cooking at home. Bananas, grapes, apples, and so forth were deliberately placed on the kitchen counter to be in easy reach for snacking. It was easier to reach for a piece of fruit than for the potato chips that were seldom stored in the kitchen pantry. Of course, there were crackers, Oreos, cheese, and good old oatmeal raisin cookies that I totally enjoyed. Juices and water served to quench the thirst, and they were kept cool in the refrigerator. I was never a fan of prepackaged snacks and drinks. Not only were those snacks deemed to be not so healthy, but they were also expensive, especially for a family with four children.

That was Health Intelligence right there! I did not know at the time but I was merely following the path of my parents, who had provided remarkably healthy meals. Now I understand that they also were Health Intelligent. Sure, my children would indulge from time to time, when they were traveling, in little packages of Twinkies, HoHos, a CapriSun, or the little bags of potato chips or Doritos like their classmates, but when I look back at those days I realize that I was setting my children up for a healthy life.

The way my parents dealt with food during my childhood days has helped me make Health Intelligent choices as an adult. Beyond that, my parents taught me how to be creative with food in a way to which many of my peers were probably never exposed. I was given opportunity after opportunity to explore food in the kitchen and at the grocery store. I was given the freedom to experiment with food, bake cakes, and perfect stewed chicken with my mom. It was those experiences that I drew from to encourage my children to explore ethnic recipes from their Jamaican side and their American side. They learned to make dumplings, ackee (a popular Jamaican vegetable), and salted cod. To date, this is one of their favorite breakfast dishes.

Taking inventory of your food habits is not an isolated action. Rather, it should be something that you frequently think about, reflect on, and modify. The only way to become smarter and more Health Intelligent is to understand where you have been with food, how you feel about food now, and where you are going with your healthy eating habits. So, start by focusing on food.

Focus on Food

Part of healthy eating is being mindful about what you're eating and thoroughly enjoying every bite that you put into your mouth. If you're eating that delicious bowl of chocolate ice cream with your own overflowing spoonfuls of peanut butter added in, then you should not feel guilty about it. When you pair food with feelings of negativity and anxiety, eating becomes stressful, and, as you know, stressful eating is not beneficial for anyone. So you make a not-so-great food choice every now and then. That is totally allowed. What's not allowed is letting yourself feel guilty about it to the point that food is no longer something you love but something that conjures up negative feelings. We all know where that choice puts us. When we put labels on food that say that some things are better than others and some foods are unhealthy for us, then it makes sense that it might become hard to enjoy something we think is bad. We are constantly telling ourselves things such as, "I should eat more vegetables," "I should have broccoli instead of French fries," or "I should not have eaten that extra scoop." But we make choices about what we eat, and choice is a conscious function of our brain. Therefore, we should assert ourselves and positively frame our choices as purposeful: we *chose* to eat the whole bag of potato chips in one sitting. Perhaps it will not be a choice we will make again, or maybe it will be. But regardless of whether or not we outdo ourselves on the next bag, we choose it. No one is telling us if it's good or bad or what we should or should not do. We have a choice. We choose what we consume. We choose how we feel about our food experiences.

Mindful Eating

How can we be sure that we enjoy and savor everything we eat, and avoid the shame and guilt associated with indulging? It's not easy. Being mindful of each bite is meant to help prevent that kind of negativity. But that means not getting lost in the latest reality show while eating, and not eating on the fly while driving through rush hour traffic. It means sitting down at a table, watching what you eat, truly tasting it, really enjoying each bite, and even setting your fork down in between bites to ensure proper digestion and savoring. That is being mindful.

Eating mindfully is necessary for good health. For adults, eating mindfully may mean that we need to think about food in a different way than we learned to as children. If we can do this, then eating can become a positive experience that is not based on guilt, stress, worry, and overindulgence. Stressors such as holidays can signal our bodies to take in as much food as possible and store it; we may need to learn to relax around these events so we can enjoy the food we're eating. Mindfulness can help us make the most of our food choices.

In her book *The Four-Day Win: End Your Diet War and Achieve Thinner Peace*, life coach Martha Beck offered the following straightforward ways to be more mindful of what you are eating:

1. Get in touch with the sensory gratification and feelings of love and togetherness that food evokes.
2. Give thanks! Gratitude and appreciation aren't compatible with feeling stressed. Give thanks and reflect on your food and stress will be gone.

3. All food is good. Remove the idea that some food is good and some food is bad. Judging your food becomes stressful and results in emotional eating.
4. When you feel frustrated, guilty, ashamed, or angry after eating the whole bag, replay the situation. This time, enjoy each and every bite, savoring the flavor.
5. Enjoy what's on your plate. Never eat anything you do not enjoy, and enjoy everything you eat—be mindful.

When it comes to comfort foods that are not so healthy, such as fattening desserts, a little goes a long way. Research suggests that after a few bites your senses start to become dulled. You'll actually have a more intense and pleasurable experience with sweets if you take no more than four bites. A week later you'll recall the experience with as much pleasure as if you had polished off the whole thing. So have a few bites of chocolate cake, then set it aside, and you'll get equal the pleasure with lower cost.

Indulge a little, be satisfied, and stop before it's excessive and unnecessary. That is mindful eating. Being fully conscious, aware, and mindful of your eating can help you make better choices to keep your eating in control and will help prevent overeating.

Choice and Control

We have a thousand choices every day, and we can decide whether to use our knowledge to make our choices. Instinctively, we probably already know whether the consequence of a choice is going to be a good or bad. With eating, the choice to use our Health Intelligence becomes just as critical as using any of the other multiple intelligences in situations where they are relevant. We may know how to be interpersonally appropriate with others, know all the social mores and rules, and understand the flow of society and why we should behave certain ways, but unless we actually choose to behave in ways that avoid shame and punishment and are consistent with personal integrity, we're not making full use of our interpersonal intelligence. Then what's the point of having it? The same goes for using Health Intelligence in our eating choices.

Rather than originating entirely in either nature or nurture, intelligence is a combination of the two. Certainly, as previously noted, everyone is born with some level of each intelligence, however limited or expansive. Experiences, family, choices, friends, biology, and a million other things can determine how each type of intelligence is nurtured, strengthened, or minimized. It's possible to assess an individual's intelligence profile, but it's less important to know what our personal levels are in each area than it is to learn how to support, nurture, and expand our various intelligences so that each is being used to its maximum capacity.

We make choices every day. With each choice, we have the opportunity to make small changes that can end up having a substantial impact on personal health. For example, I can choose to go meatless for one day each week. It may not seem like a big deal, but eliminating fat and calories and the other negatives associated with meat can make a difference. I can choose to try low-fat or fat-free options; sometimes it's easy to adopt the substitute for health benefits and sometimes the taste is just not the same. You can easily cut out the fat where you can and keep the full-fat variety of your favorites. I might not like the way fat-free crackers taste, so I'll stick with the original version, but I can swap out full-fat sour cream for the fat-free alternative without sacrificing much of the flavor.

Part of the trick in making better choices about food is making sure that you are serving and eating the correct portion size. If you read the nutritional label, it may surprise you how different the portions are from what you normally consume. I can choose to consume the recommended portion size (the company has conveniently supplied me with that information), or I can choose to disregard the recommendation. I can choose to eat the whole bag, or I can choose to eat a third of the bag and then put it away.

Perfect Portions

Research has repeatedly shown that when people are given large portions, they eat more.

There's a rationale for this. When you eat out, you want as much as you can get for your money. After all, food is expensive. When you purchase food, it seems like the bigger the container, the better. Thirty percent more in the package means a better value. When you're at a party with food, you can always go back for seconds and thirds. More is better, right?

This may have been true a hundred years ago when starvation was a real possibility. Times have changed. Most of us have access to more food than we need—in fact, you could say that we each have access to a toxic amount of food. Today, just because food is available and put in front of you does not mean you have to eat it all in one sitting. You can choose to take half of the meal home for tomorrow's lunch. You can choose to portion out your food or measure your food when you eat it. You can choose not to return to the buffet table for extras. There are always choices about portions.

An interesting study by Sidney Fry in 2012 showed how people tend to over-consume without even knowing it. Researchers found that:

1. Ninety percent of people over-poured cereal past the recommended one-cup measurement of a daily serving for 120 calories.
2. People poured an average of 3 2/3 cup, which increased the potential calorie intake to 440.
3. Only 25% of Americans actually eat five or more servings of vegetables every day (one serving is half a cup).

Portion control is not easy, especially when it's food we enjoy. Would you like to trick yourself into changing how much you eat? You can! You can choose to literally downsize your plates at home, because if you use smaller eight-inch plates you can actually eat less than you would with a big thirteen-inch plate. Change the composition of what's on your plate too. Cover most of the plate with vegetables or fruit and add in protein and grain as a side dish, not the other way around, as many of us were raised to do. Although we may have been trained to join the clean-plate club, it's wise to keep a portion of the meal on your plate and turn the food into leftovers for tomorrow, feed it to the dog, or compost it. The less food consumed—especially if you are not really hungry—the healthier you will feel.

Indulge in Moderation

Even if you're full at the end of the meal and you're offered dessert (or you have been trained from childhood to want dessert), you have the choice to eat it or not. You can choose to eat it now, later, or in a smaller portion. Whatever you choose, you should not feel as if you have to deprive yourself. People might say, "Don't skimp on dessert." Who would want to? Using Health Intelligence doesn't mean you have to deprive yourself of dessert or other indulgences.

It's easy to make instant desserts that contain fruit, yogurt, or other sweetly satisfying meal conclusions. Desserts are meant to cleanse the palate and leave you feeling full and finished, not wanting more. There are plenty of filling choices. It's all about being mindful of what you choose.

If we deprive ourselves of certain foods, we feel we have missed out on something that our body is craving. We should allow ourselves to satisfy that need in moderation so that we do not feel deprived. We can certainly make smarter choices with what we indulge in as well. We can choose low-fat or fat-free options, or we can choose a smaller portion size. These choices mean we can enjoy what we love without the guilt and extra weight gain.

In this fast-paced world, people might claim that we do not have time to enjoy what we eat, but we can choose to do so. We must use our power to take control of our eating. The blame should not be placed on fast food restaurants, consumer packaging that lured us in, or the latest craze in prepared meals. We only have ourselves to blame for the choices we make. If life is moving too fast, we need to make choices to slow it down. One of the best ways to make things easier and slow them down is to keep it simple.

Keep It Simple

Simple! It's all about eating simply. Go back to basics (raw, natural, and organic) and as fresh as fresh can get. That is the best way to ensure that you are eating healthily. Of course, making choices for things such as lean meat and darker green vegetables are better than some of the alternatives, but generally the most basic foods are the healthiest. It's hard to go wrong if you're eating natural foods that are prepared without a lot of extras. If you have never eaten a raw green bean, you should certainly try it. They are delicious, and I even find it difficult to eat them cooked because I simply love the taste of them raw. Cucumbers with a pinch of sea salt are delicious. Tomatoes with a little balsamic vinegar and fresh mozzarella are delicious. Fresh summer peaches at peak ripeness are simply perfect. A crunchy Honeycrisp apple is amazing. There are so many choices that are delicious as they are, raw and uncensored. If you have not tried vegetables and fruits this way, it would be a great exercise in expanding your palette—and that of your children, who of course are watching what you do.

The same notion of keeping it simple applies to grains as well. If you're eating whole grains, then you're consuming all the best parts of the grain rather than just a portion of it as in processed or refined products. White flour, white bread, white rice, and pasta are refined products that are less nutritious than whole grains. Look for whole grains such as oat, buckwheat, whole wheat, bran, corn, brown rice, rye, and quinoa, to name just a few. Look for grain products where the first item on the label reads "whole wheat," "whole meal," or "whole corn," and you will be getting something that is as close to natural as possible.

The idea of keeping it simple applies to the protein group too. This group includes meat, chicken, seafood, fish, beans, nuts, seeds, eggs, tofu, and soy-based products. Proteins should always be fresh and handled correctly to avoid contamination of other foods. It's important to avoid consuming raw meats or their juices. All preparation areas should be thoroughly cleaned after contact with raw meat to kill salmonella and other bacteria. Additionally, consumers should read all package directions about how to store, thaw, and prepare foods appropriately. For additional tips on meat and protein safety, visit choosemyplate.gov/food-groups/protein-foods-tips.html.

Proteins that are prepared with minimal additional ingredients are best. Keep it simple: a little salt, a little pepper, or a little olive oil can help enhance the natural flavors. It also makes perfect sense that low-fat or lean meats are better than meats with higher fat content. If you see fat on your meat, cut it off before preparing it and choose a method of cooking that does not include extra oils or butters (for example, poaching or broiling). Processed meats such as deli lunchmeats, hams, hot dogs, canned meats, or pre-seasoned roasts often have added sodium content that is unnecessary. It's better to stay away from those kinds of processed meats, or at least eat them infrequently. If you do enjoy those kinds of meats, choose low-fat or low-sodium. Nuts and seeds are often flavored with salt as well, so making the choice of the lightly salted or unsalted variety is a good idea. In choosing fish or other seafood, the best selections are those that are high in omega 3 fatty acids such as salmon or trout.

Keeping it simple is a lot easier than you might think. The dairy group is no exception. Choose fat-free or low-fat milk or soy-based milk products. You might even choose products that have been fortified with extra calcium. You can find low-fat yogurt, low-fat sour cream, low-fat cottage cheese, and a variety of other fat-free or reduced-fat dairy products. Dairy products should be handled, stored, and prepared appropriately to ensure the healthiest outcome. For example, raw eggs should be kept away from other foods. Preparing eggs without extra butter and cheese is a healthy way to serve them.

Simple eating is not difficult. It may take a bit of practice, especially for the individual who likes to add lots of extras to his or her food such as extra butter, extra cheese, or extra sauce. If you are one of those people, challenge yourself to start by using less of the extras. Cut down the way you indulge in those extras and make your way back to simple and basic in a gradual way that will not shock your system and make you feel deprived of the things you love. Pay attention to what you are eating, thoroughly enjoy it, and continue to keep it simple.

It's hard to keep track of all the changes in nutrition and healthy eating. It's easy to get confused about what's healthy and what's not. One day the media tells you that eggs are good for you, and the next day they pose a cholesterol problem. The same is true many other kinds of foods and beverages. So, how can we be sure that what we are eating is right? Well, we can use our Health Intelligence and keep it simple. We can read the latest research, and we can continue to eat what we eat, just in moderation. Nobody should drastically alter their diet based on the latest food fad. Research is ongoing and will change rapidly. There is no sense in making ridiculous changes; unless you're at the point where drastic changes are needed for your well being, go ahead and make small ones that are barely noticeable in your daily routine.

Chapter 14

Recipe for a Healthy Lifestyle

A healthy body is a guest-chamber for
the soul; a sick body is a prison.
— Francis Bacon

So far, this book has focused on societal problems associated with eating and overeating as well as how various institutions (such as media, family, and schools) influence our everyday eating habits. A healthy lifestyle begins with proper care of the physical body, including eating and drinking foods and beverages with appropriate nutritional content. Ultimately, your eating habits are up to you. You have control over what you eat and you have some control over what others (especially your children) eat. Maybe obesity and overeating are not a problem for you or your family; perhaps you just want to be healthier. We can all stand to be a little healthier. If you want to improve the good eating habits you already have, there are several easy ways to make changes that may not be noticeable to you every day, but which can make a dramatic impact on your future.

Top Ten Healthy Eating Strategies

Every day we're told about some new secret to a healthy life, and it can be difficult to keep up with the changes in food trends and figure out what actually works. But regardless of your eating history or your goals for your eating habits there are timeless strategies that can be applied across the board. The following are the basics that are general, simple, and easy to apply to any current lifestyle.

1. Eat when you're hungry, not for recreation.
2. Minimize portions.
3. Eat natural, flavorful foods. Enjoy every bite!
4. Eat mindfully and intelligently.
5. Focus on the food when you are eating, not on the television.
6. Diversify your diet.
7. Shop smart.
8. Don't deprive yourself—eat a little bit of everything.
9. Indulge occasionally.
10. Use food-free self-rewards.

The overall takeaway of this list is to be more conscious of what you are eating. When you increase your awareness of everyday habits, they can be much easier to analyze and modify. If you learn to listen to your body, you will know when you are hungry, when you are not, why you eat what you do, how feelings affect when and what you eat, and how you can start making other small changes to improve overall health. Increased awareness is the basis for healing and growth.

Top Ten Grocery Shopping Strategies

Obviously, grocery shopping plays an extremely important part in healthy eating. Most of us shop at least once or twice a week. We're always running to the store to grab that jug of milk, a loaf of bread, or the one item that's missing from the recipe we want to cook for dinner. Large chain grocery stores are great because they have almost everything you could ever imagine in every flavor, in every size, and in many different brands. But these stores have made it difficult to avoid temptation. If you're like me, you probably go shopping for a list of items and return home with a trunk full of unnecessary (but tasty) items that you just *had* to have. The following simple strategies can help focus your grocery shopping on the right kinds of choices—healthy choices—with a few indulgent items.

1. Never grocery shop when you're hungry.
2. Choose something new and healthy each time.
3. Read and compare nutrition labels.
4. Choose one specialty item (for example, ethnic food, sauces, and spices).
5. Splurge a little (for example, quinoa pasta, Kobe beef, or a gourmet cheese).
6. Stock up on kitchen staples (for example, tuna, beans, pasta, and rice).
7. Plan ahead and shop for the whole week (consider what to do with leftovers).
8. Focus on fresh (fill the cart with fruits and veggies).
9. Choose in-season produce for the best flavor.
10. Look for prepared shortcuts (for example, chicken, tuna, breads, and proteins).

Some of these strategies may seem obvious, but I know that it takes discipline and practice not to get sucked into putting goodies that are not really good for you into your cart. Changing your shopping habits does not have to be difficult. Start with a well-planned list, make room for your splurge item, and focus on healthy food. We do not always have time to read nutrition labels, but if you focus on one product type each time you shop, soon you'll learn which product is best for you. Being aware of new options and new shortcut ideas can cut down on shopping and cooking time and can help keep you focused on healthy choices.

Top Six Foods That Fight Fat

Some people focus on the fat and calorie content when they think of food. It's only natural; we've been programmed to be conscious of weight and the foods that pack on the pounds. We continue to look for ways to cut the fat from our diets so that we can be healthier. There is a plethora of information about healthy eating and how to fight fat. Here are six simple foods that can be incorporated into your diet to help fight fat:

1. Nuts. Fiber keeps you full.
2. Fat-free milk. As calcium increases, body fat decreases.
3. Oatmeal. It helps curb your appetite.
4. Green tea. It boosts your metabolism.
5. Vegetable juice. Drink it before meals and you will eat fewer calories.
6. Eggs. Eating them early in the day means you will eat less throughout the day.

These foods can be helpful in combating the negative effects of other foods, and many of these foods are on the list of healthy foods to add to your diet anyway. Adding them to your diet is easy. There is instant oatmeal, mini packets of nuts, lots of easy ways to prepare eggs, flavored green tea in cold and hot varieties, and prepared vegetable juices that taste like fruit juice.

Healthy Eating Strategies by Food Group

Overall eating strategies can serve as a general guide, but sometimes we want to make more specific changes in the way we eat. The next few strategies include more detailed ways that we can modify our choices within each of the five food groups as well as some other specific strategies.

Proteins

- ✓ Substitute lean meats for full fat meats.
- ✓ Use beans, tofu, fish, and other proteins more often.
- ✓ A three-ounce portion of meat is about the size of the palm of your hand; a portion the size of your thumb is one ounce.
- ✓ Get enough protein (for example, fish, poultry, lean meat, eggs, yogurt, cottage cheese, nuts, and lean meats) because a protein-rich diet will help your exercise plan because protein revs up your metabolism.
- ✓ Check the sodium level, especially in processed meats such as lunchmeat or ham.

Fruits and Vegetables

- ✓ Eat five to nine servings per day of colorful vegetables and fruits.

- ✓ Focus on super foods (for example, blueberries, acai and goji berries, nuts, and beans).
- ✓ Add one salad per day to increase vegetable intake.
- ✓ Make smoothies and drink your daily servings of fruit.
- ✓ Add a slice of lemon to your water to help curb your appetite.
- ✓ Add some broccoli to your diet to protect your heart and help your eyesight.
- ✓ Consume some citrus to fight cancer.
- ✓ Leafy greens are good for your eyes.
- ✓ When cooking vegetables, do not boil out the nutrients; microwave, steam, or go raw instead. Boiled broccoli retains only half of its Vitamin C, whereas steamed broccoli retains up to one hundred percent.

Dairy

- ✓ Milk may help prevent colon cancer.
- ✓ Try low-fat, fat-free, or soy milk.
- ✓ Choose active-culture yogurt to maintain healthy bacteria in the gut.
- ✓ Focus on whole grain products.
- ✓ Wheat bran is good for regularity.
- ✓ Buy brown rice (be mindful to wash it multiple times prior to cooking to rid it of possibly harmful arsenic), crackers, multigrain bread, and other grain products. White variations mean they have been more processed and have lost some nutrients.

Other Food Strategies

- ✓ Enjoy some dark chocolate for its antioxidant benefits.
- ✓ Use good fats such as avocado, nuts, olives, fish, and veggies.
- ✓ Use olive oil instead of vegetable oil to increase consumption of good fats.
- ✓ Choose red wine to help lower heart disease risk and boost good cholesterol.
- ✓ Drink tea (especially green teas) to fight viruses.
- ✓ Consume high-fiber foods to cut your blood pressure and fight hypertension.
- ✓ Measure and eat the correct serving size.
- ✓ Keep some fats in your diet. Good fats trigger gene activity in the liver, which spurs metabolism.
- ✓ When you're watching what you eat, it's okay to snack on calcium-rich foods, fiber-rich foods, or naturally sweet and low-calorie fruit. You should not feel hungry during a diet.
- ✓ Focus on your food. Snacking in front of the television leads to excessive recreational eating.
- ✓ Eliminate sugary drinks, including juice, and replace them with water, non-caloric beverages, and low-fat or skim milk.
- ✓ Restrict calories enough to produce mild negative energy balance.
- ✓ Reduce intake of saturated fats, salty snacks, and high-glycemic foods, including candy, white bread, white rice, pasta, and potatoes.
- ✓ Create a balanced diet containing vegetables, fruits, whole grains, nuts, fiber, lean meat, fish, and low-fat dairy products.

Recipes

One of the best parts about eating is finding new foods to enjoy. Recipes should be used not so much as rigid instructions to follow but as opportunities for inspiration and creativity. If you look in most cookbooks or magazines, you'll find lots of really great recipes. Too often, however, there is at least one random ingredient that you have neither heard of nor have in your cupboard—things like sesame oil, shallots, rice noodles, fresh lime, garam masala, fish sauce, and ricotta cheese. While the recipe may sound delicious and the picture might look awesome, bringing together all the ingredients is just not always realistic. It's too much work, too expensive, and too time-consuming. For sure, it's not a recipe for a hurried weeknight meal. (I must note that, more and more, the food shows are putting together good recipes that are quickly and easily prepared.)

Relax! You can take nearly any recipe and modify it based on what you have available. For example, you can make an awesome Pad Thai without fish sauce or fresh lime. Cooking should be fun, not difficult. If you're on the path to becoming a culinary genius, then you can follow the recipes without wavering from the ingredient list; but for the amateur, meals should be easy and straightforward.

It's worth repeating that recipes should be used as *inspiration*. The experience of cooking should be infused with creative freedom. One easy way to incorporate new foods into your cooking is to take a staple that you love—a comfort food—and have more fun with it. Be creative. Look at what you have in the pantry or fridge and try a new combination. This is the spirit behind the following suggestions, which are not actually recipes, but can provide some inspiration for new meal favorites.

Macaroni and Cheese

Children love macaroni and cheese. It's always better to make it from scratch as opposed to using the boxed mixture. However, whether you make it from the box or from scratch, there are endless ways to change up macaroni and cheese to make it new and exciting. To make your own basic cheese sauce, do the following:

In a saucepan, melt 4 tablespoons of butter and 2 tablespoons of flour and mix well. Add 1 cup of milk and 2 cups of your favorite cheeses (American melts well). Pour the sauce over any kind of cooked noodles and bake at 350 degrees for 30 minutes or until the cheese starts to brown.

You can also apply the following variations:

1. Make it fiesta style by adding tomato chunks, olives, sweet corn, chicken pieces, spicy cheese, and beans, and serve it on a bed of lettuce.
2. Add tater tots, ground beef, tomatoes, pickles, mustard, and ketchup to make cheeseburger pasta.
3. Try different kinds of cheese such as goat cheese, provolone, ricotta, or blue cheese.
4. Add canned tuna fish, chopped onions, cream of mushroom soup, and green olives to make a quick tuna casserole.
5. Add different vegetables such as carrots, edamame beans (green soybeans), green beans, or peas.
6. Try Mark Bittman's Sweet Potato Chili Mac, which features the fabulously nutritious sweet potato, chipotle chile, Mexican chorizo, green onions, and cilantro.
7. Bittman's Steak House Side Mac and Cheese includes creamed spinach, sautéed mushrooms, bacon chunks, and blue cheese dressing made with Greek yogurt.

Fresh Green Salads

Salads are an easy staple to add to any diet, and the choices of what to add to a salad are endless. You can experiment with different kinds of lettuce and a variety of different vegetables, toppings, and dressings. Each new ingredient you add can change the entire flavor of the salad so you never feel as if you're eating the same old thing over and over. You can try the following suggestions:

1. Add seasonal vegetables. If corn is in season, cook it, slice it off the cob, and add it to your salad.
2. Try frozen chick peas, sweet corn, beans, or other frozen products.
3. Add some dried fruit such as cranberries, blueberries, or mango slices, or add fresh fruit such as plums, pears, or apple slices.
4. Experiment with different kinds of cheeses such as blue cheese, feta, cottage cheese, or goat cheese.
5. Add different kinds of protein such as beans, tofu, nuts, salami, pepperoni, ham, turkey, shrimp, or tuna.
6. Top your salad with crumbled crackers, Doritos, or your favorite potato chips (be careful not to use too much).
7. Make your own quick dressing. Try sour cream, garlic salt, pepper, and a touch of vinegar, or try vinegar and maple syrup with a squirt of lemon.
8. Make a fresh kale salad. Wash the kale, chop off the stalks, slice the kale, or shred into little pieces. Place in a large bowl. Drizzle with one tablespoon olive oil and ½ teaspoon of salt and sprinkle on some pepper. Then, massage the kale with your hands for 6-7 minutes until tender. Top with tomatoes, onions, cottage cheese, or whatever you like. Kale is a super food with lots of nutrients!

Stir Fry

The options for stir fry are endless as well. You can use any kind of meats, proteins, vegetables, and a variety of different seasonings. You can use whole grain rice, white rice, or noodles. Try soba noodles, which are made with buckwheat; Udon noodles, which are made with wheat; rice noodles; or whole grain pasta.

Here are some handy tips for making delicious stir fry meals:

1. Stir fry is great with the basics such as carrots, celery, onions, cabbage, broccoli, peppers, beans, snap peas, mushrooms, and bean sprouts.
2. Add in some Chinese vegetables such as bok choy, snow peas, water chestnuts, baby corn, green onions, or edamame beans.
3. Mix rice with different flavored soups, sauces, or spices. Try curry, cumin, garlic, ginger, red pepper, or a new spice you have never tried before.
4. Serve alongside different kinds of protein such as shrimp, crab meat, chicken, fish, beef, fried egg, or tofu. Tofu takes on the flavor of whatever you cook, so make the flavor more fun with your spices.
5. Make a Pad Thai version by adding chopped peanuts and bean sprouts with a squeeze of lime juice on top.

Meatloaf

Some people love meatloaf and grew up eating it the way mom made it. Maybe it was garnished with tomato sauce or a cream of mushroom sauce with some breadcrumbs, but whatever mom did to it, the recipe was consistent and filling. Here are a few new ways to try an old favorite:

1. Top your meatloaf with different kinds of cheese, onions, and fresh sliced tomatoes.
2. Top with mashed sweet potatoes.
3. Mix your ground meat with different kinds of canned soup for a new meatloaf flavor. Mix in different kinds of cheeses; try blue cheese for a "black and blue" meatloaf.
4. Try different kinds of breadcrumbs, panko crumbs, crushed potato chips, pretzels, or different flavored cracker crumbs.
5. Mix your meat with peas, lima beans, corn, carrots, or whatever vegetables you have on hand.
6. Switch up the ground beef and use ground turkey or ground lamb.
7. Slice up the meatloaf into little cubes and serve your square meatballs over spaghetti.
8. Try vegetable "meatloaf." It's made with red and green bell peppers, mushrooms, asparagus, red onion, walnuts, cheese, eggs, and a few other basic ingredients. Find the full recipe here: http://www.myrecipes.com/recipe/vegetable-meat-loaf-50400000119679

Potatoes

Potatoes are all-time favorites that appeal to both children and adults. They're hearty, filling, satisfying, and one of the most comforting of all comfort foods. Like the previous recipes, potatoes are versatile, and the options for preparing them are endless. In many recipes you can replace the regular potato with sweet potato.

1. Skillet fry potato chunks with olive oil, garlic salt, and black pepper. Top with sour cream and cheese. Add taco seasoning for a fiesta flavor.
2. Try baked potatoes with a variety of toppings, but avoid adding big hunks of fat such as butter or margarine. Include reasonable amounts of cheese, sour cream, or plain yogurt. You can also add tomatoes or broccoli.
3. Roast sliced potatoes with zucchini, carrots, eggplant, and squash.
4. Mash and mix the potatoes with cheese, seafood, or whatever vegetables you like.
5. Make the basic cheese sauce described in the macaroni and cheese section. Pour over diced potatoes, and then add peas, corn, or any other vegetables to make a cheesy potato and vegetable casserole.
6. Make potato pancakes and serve them with cottage cheese or apple sauce.
7. Serve potatoes with eggs, salmon or ham, and vegetables in a breakfast omelet.
8. Try Potato and Root Vegetable Mashers, which are a mix of sweet potatoes and turnips. Find the full recipe at http://www.myrecipes.com/recipe/potato-root-vegetable-mashers-50400000119694/.
9. Try Cajun Stuffed Potatoes, which feature yellow onion, green bell peppers, celery, red pepper, and crawfish meat. Find the full recipe at http://www.myrecipes.com/ recipe/ cajun-stuffed-potatoes-50400000119696/

Sandwiches

Sandwiches are another staple that many people eat almost every day. How can we make the typical sandwich a little more fun and exciting? Sub shops are always trying to find new and exciting ways to dress up meats and cheeses, and we can steal a few ideas from the shops we love and make the same sandwiches at home.

1. Start with your favorite meats, but don't be afraid to try new meat combinations. Use leftover turkey or chicken for your sandwich. Try tuna fish or canned chicken made into tuna or chicken salad with a few tablespoons of sour cream or mayonnaise and some seasoning. How about a shrimp sandwich? Leftover pork? Pulled pork? Ham? Try some new meats and proteins.
2. Cheese is another favorite part of any sandwich. Try new cheeses (for example, provolone, cheddar, American, brie, ricotta, Muenster, Co-jack, or any other kind). Try two or three kinds of cheese on the same sandwich.
3. Use whole grain bread, a hoagie bun, a tortilla, ciabatta bread, whole grain crackers, or an English muffin instead of plain white bread.
4. Add lettuce. Try the many different kinds of lettuce that are available beyond the iceberg variety including Boston, radicchio, bibb, spinach, Swiss chard, romaine, butterhead, arugula, endive, and kale.
5. Try something different and add sliced cabbage, bean sprouts, onion, tomato, cucumber, peppers, or something you have never tried on a sandwich before.
6. Think of combinations that might taste good together.

How about pear, prosciutto, and brie? How about apples, provolone, and ham?

7. Try a side of sweet potato chips, veggie chips, blue corn chips, or quinoa chips.
8. Instead of mustard or mayonnaise, garnish with hummus or plain Greek yogurt.

Pizza

Pizza is obviously another favorite for children and adults. Part of its appeal may be that there are so many different ways to prepare pizza with different sauces, toppings, meats, and vegetables. There is something for everyone when it comes to pizza. Contrary to what some people might think, pizza is actually very easy to make at home. It's inexpensive and you can probably make it yourself faster than the pizza place can deliver it. You can make a homemade crust or you can buy your favorite premade crust (for example, Boboli and Martha White).

Easy pizza crust. Use 1 package of yeast dissolved in 1 cup of warm water, 2 ½ cups of flour, and 2 tablespoons of olive oil. Mix well and let stand for 10 minutes to rise. Roll out, poke with fork, place in pan, precook for 3 minutes, and then, top with toppings and cook for 8-10 minutes at 450 degrees.

Switch up the toppings and try new combinations, such as spinach and feta cheese, mushroom and goat cheese, ground beef and blue cheese, chicken and Mexican cheese mix.

Try new vegetables such as red peppers, green peppers, banana peppers, fresh tomato slices, black and green olives, onions, spinach, mushrooms, or potato slices.

Try different kinds of meat including turkey sausage, ground turkey, chicken, and barbecue flavored chicken.

Try a variety of cheeses such as mozzarella, provolone, ricotta, parmesan, goat cheese, blue cheese, Mexican-flavored cheeses, Colby, Jalapeño cheddar, and white cheddar.

Change it up and add fruit like pineapple chunks, pear or plum slices, or dried mangos.

Gyro pizza. Use basic pizza crust, top with cooked ground lamb, tomatoes, onions, and cheese. After the pizza is cooked, top with a mix of sour cream, chopped cucumber, and garlic salt.

Soup

Soup is another staple, especially during the cold winter months. It's easy to make a large batch that will last the entire week, and you can freeze a portion so it will last a few weeks longer. There are soups with all kinds of bases and broth as starters, including chicken broth, beef broth, vegetable broth, cream, and tomato. Depending on what flavors you like, there are endless possibilities when it comes to making this one-pot meal.

Start with a basic broth of water and some spices, a prepared broth, or a simple canned soup such as cream of chicken. Beware of prepared broths that are very high in sodium—you're always better off adding your own salt to taste. To the base add your own combinations of vegetables, proteins, and grains.

Slice up your favorite vegetables or some that you have never tried before. Use frozen vegetables for a shortcut to quick soup. Try celery, carrots, beans, cabbage, onions, peas, corn, okra, potatoes, sweet potatoes, and broccoli.

Add protein such as chicken chunks, beef cubes, lean ground meatballs, tofu, or different kinds of beans.

Experiment with different spices without adding too much salt. Let the flavors of the vegetables and proteins come through.

Add some well-washed rice or noodles such as ditalini pasta or bite-sized choochoo wheels.

Make your own butter dumplings. In a bowl, mix 4 tablespoons of butter, 1 egg, and 6 tablespoons of whole wheat flour. Season as you wish and drop into boiling soup. Cook until the dumplings rise to the top.

Farina dumplings. In a bowl, beat 1 egg (warmed to room temperature), add 2 tablespoons of melted butter, and gradually add ½ cup of farina until thick. Season as you wish. Drop into boiling soup and cook until they rise to the top.

Have Fun With Food

Play your own version of The Food Network's *Chopped*—the personalized edition, without the judging. Let's say you have a few random ingredients left in your pantry or cupboards, and you have no idea what you can make for dinner.

Challenge yourself. What can you make with zucchini, arugula, strawberries, and tortilla wraps? How about zucchini-arugula salad with strawberry vinaigrette and tortilla strip croutons; mashed zucchini and strawberry arugula wraps; or tortilla pizza topped with strawberry-arugula salad and zucchini salsa? The choices are only as limited as your imagination. You might actually enjoy what you made. You might even invent a new favorite recipe combo.

Stack Up on Staples

The more resourceful you are, the sooner you will learn to shop like a professional. You'll know what items you can count on as go-to items that can act as a base for a variety of different meals. You'll shop in a way that will give you a more versatile appetite. If you always have beans, you can always make something that is based in a solid protein. If you always have tortilla wraps, you'll always have some sort of quick sandwich option. If you always have tuna, you can make tuna salad, tuna casserole, or tuna whatever. You can grow to know what staple ingredients you need to keep in your pantry. For me, it's some type of whole wheat pasta noodles, taco seasoning, a variety of frozen vegetables, beans, salmon, chicken breast, canned tuna fish, and a lot of fresh salad mixtures; that way, I've always got something to work with to build my meal from and to create the next "that's my new favorite meal" winning combination.

Use Shortcuts

Shortcuts are an easy way to make a tasty meal in no time. There is no shame in making a meal that is tasty and fast and not entirely made from scratch. Companies spend millions of dollars and tons of time coming up with quick products, so we should use whatever is available to us to make our lives easier. Just remember to use your Health Intelligence and read the labels carefully!

- ✓ Stop off and get a pre-roasted chicken or a bucket of grilled chicken; use it for your chicken salad, tacos, or homemade chicken soup.
- ✓ Cook up some boxed macaroni and cheese or rice and add your own vegetables and proteins.

- ✓ Buy the bagged lettuce to start your salad. After thoroughly washing the lettuce in cool water, add shredded carrots and grape tomatoes for a quick salad.
- ✓ Buy your favorite bag of Doritos and arrange them on a microwaveable plate. Top with shredded cheese, and microwave for 45 seconds to one minute. Add diced tomato, diced onions, chopped olives, diced peppers, refried beans, ground meat, or whatever else you choose for instant nachos.
- ✓ Buy basic chocolate or vanilla ice cream or frozen yogurt. Top with peanut butter, candy pieces, cereal pieces, or fruit to make your own sundaes.
- ✓ Buy your favorite vegetables and fruits to make that tasty smoothie.

Sharing Health Intelligence

One of the most powerful things about healthy eating is that you can share your tricks and wisdom with others. Once you've learned a recipe that your family loves, or you've tried something new and found the value in it, you can pass on your wisdom to others, including your children, your friends, your neighbors, and other members of your family.

We can also use the wisdom of others who have used their own Health Intelligence to provide us with valuable information. Magazines, books, online resources, blogs, and dieticians can provide us with brilliant ideas that are meant to be shared and used. We can learn from others who have experimented with food and nutrition, and we should continue to turn to these resources for information. For example, *Nutrition Action* magazine is a terrific resource for nutrition information and comparison shopping. Each edition features several categories of foods (for example, frozen yogurt, bread, and cheese) and reveals the products that are nutritionally best and worst in each category. The authors compare calories, fats, and other important nutritional aspects, and then provide the reader with a sorted list of products. The nice thing about *Nutrition Action* is that the resource is small, compact, and direct with its presentation of facts and research. It's easy to read and very straightforward, so it takes a lot of the guesswork out of shopping based on nutritional value.

Lots of information is readily available to the consumer, and most of it is free. We should use it!

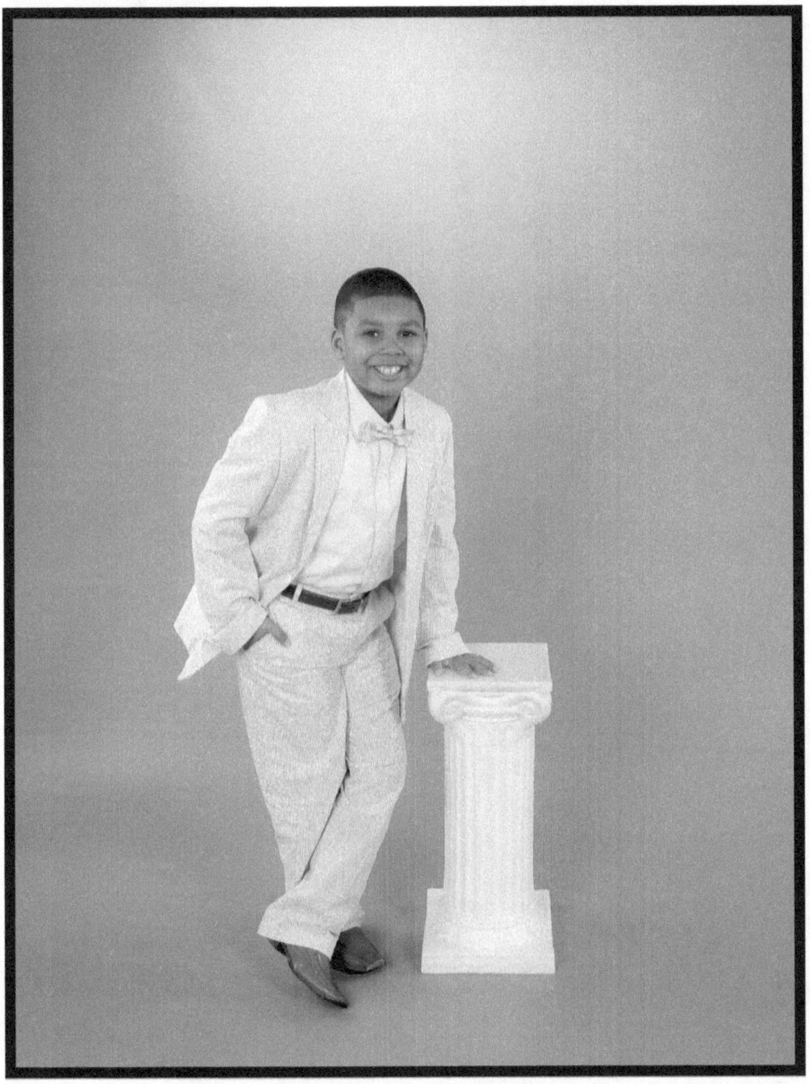

Benjamin, an autism survivor.
Education is the key to giving every child a chance.

CHAPTER 15

It's Time to Begin

He who has health, has hope. And he
who has hope, has everything.
— Arabian proverb

Beginning a journey toward better health is a process of changing one small habit at a time. Making small and gradual changes will allow you time to practice new ways of doing things without throwing your world into a tailspin. If you do this, you'll experience a paradigm shift in the way you think about food, life, relationships, and spiritual growth.

What is a habit? It's the result of combining knowledge (what to do), skill (how to do), and desire (want to do). In his bestselling book *The Seven Habits of Highly Effective People*, author Stephen R. Covey revealed how we can all be more effective in business, family, friendships, school, and other aspects of life if we follow his seven habits, which can easily be applied to Health Intelligence as well:

1. Be proactive. Make conscious choices and responses.
2. Begin with the end in mind. Start with a clear understanding of your goal destination so you can better understand where you are now and if you are on the right path to get there.

3. Put first things first. Prioritize, organize, and remain disciplined as you speed toward your goals.
4. Think win/win. Seek mutual learning, mutual influence, and mutual benefits.
5. Seek first to understand, then to be understood. You gain knowledge that you can share with others in a credible, understandable way.
6. Synergize. The whole is greater than the sum of its parts. Work together.
7. Sharpen the saw. Renew the physical, spiritual, mental, and socio-emotional aspects of life.

When we're thinking of making any form of life change including improving our Health Intelligence, keep the seven habits in mind: they will help propel you forward and will keep you on track to achieve satisfactory results. The seven habits are easy to understand, globally applicable, and keep the focus on multiple working parts that require attention. This kind of structure can be helpful in achieving our personal health goals.

One of the most fundamental aspects of constructive change in the life of an individual is having the ability to create a balance. By balancing the four dimensions of our nature—physical, mental, spiritual, and socio-emotional—we're able to attain and maintain a more fulfilled life. Covey identified the need for balance in maintaining the four aforementioned areas, and suggested that neglecting one area affects the rest. Similarly, improving in one area can increase one's abilities in other areas. The four dimensions are interdependent, and can affect one another in drastic ways. We should keep all of these areas fresh, healthy, and alive through a process of renewal. Covey suggested that personal growth is like an upward spiral which requires us to learn, commit, and advance to higher planes of success.

Health Intelligence requires the same kind of process, beginning with knowledge, skill, and desire. If we know what to do, how to do it, and have the desire to achieve, positive results will happen. Yes, we can do it. The bottom line is that with determination we can change. We can become more Health Intelligent. Healthy living can become a habit.

I hope that this book has provided you with a solid foundation of knowledge about healthy eating, taking care of the four dimensions of the self, strategizing a healthier lifestyle, and learning a few basic skills to get you started on the path toward improved Health Intelligence. Finding the desire and following through with the ongoing process of learning, committing, and doing are entirely up to you. Let us all help each other to live healthier and happier lives. Let us especially help our children, so that each child can say, "I stood on the shoulder of a giant who was able to help me become Health Intelligent, and now that I understand, I'll be able to live a wholesome and healthy life, and for that I'll be forever grateful."

References and Resources

Bay State Health. (2010). *Weight loss surgery program receives high accreditation from American College of Surgeons.* Retrieved from http://www.baystatehealth.com/ Baystate/ Main+Nav/Clinical+Services/Departments/Surgery/ Weight+Loss+ Surgery +Program/Patient+Information/ Overweight+and+Obesity

Beck, M. (2007). *The four-day win: End your diet.* New York, NY: Rodale.

Beier, M. E., & Ackerman, P. L. (2003). Determinants of health knowledge: An investigation of age, gender, abilities, personality, and interests. *Journal of Personality and Social Psychology, 84*, 439-449.

Birch, L. L., & Fisher, J.O. (1998). Development of eating behaviors among children and adolescents. *Pediatrics: Official Journal of the American Academy of Pediatrics, 101*, 539.

Bittman, M. (2011). *Is junk food really cheaper?* Retrieved from http://www.nytimes .com/2011/09/25/opinion/sunday/is-junk-food-really-cheaper.html?_r=1

Bloom, B. (1956). *Bloom's taxonomy eduscapes.* Retrieved from http://www.eduscapes.com/tap/topic69.htm

Boyce, T. (2007). The media and obesity. *Obesity Reviews, 8*(Suppl. 1), 201-205.

Brooks-Gunn, J., & Duncan, G.J. (1997). The effects of poverty on children. *The Future of Children, 7*(2), 55-71.

Brown, R., & Ogden, J. (2004). Children's eating attitudes and behaviour: A study of the modelling and control theories of parental influence. *Health Education Research, 19*, 261-271.

Brown, S. L., Schiraldi, G. R., & Wrobleski, M. P. (2009). Association of eating behaviors and obesity with psychosocial and familial influences. *American Journal of Health Education, 40*(2), 80-89.

Burdette, H. L. E., & Whitaker, R. C. (2004). Neighborhood playgrounds, fast food restaurants, and crime: Relationships to overweight in low-income preschool children. *Preventive Medicine, 38*, 57-63.

Casey, P. H., Simpson, P. M., Gossett, J. M., Bogle, J., Champagne, C. M., Connell, C., . . . Weber, J. (2006). The association of child and household food insecurity with childhood overweight status. *Pediatrics, 118*, 1406. Retrieved from http://www .pediatrics.aappublications.org/content/118/5/e1406.full.pdf

Cohen, H. Y. (2012). *What is intelligence and how is it measured?* Retrieved from http://www.aboutintelligence.co.uk/what-intelligence.html

Covey, S. R. (1989). *The Seven Habits of Highly Effective People.* New York< NY: Fireside.

Cutler, D. M., & Lleras-Muney, A. (2007). *Education and health.* Ann Arbor, MI:

Nutritional Policy Center.

Deckelbaum, R. J., & Williams, C. L. (2001). Childhood obesity: The health issue. *Obesity Research, 9,* S239-S243.

Doghramji, K. (2005). The effects of alcohol on sleep. Medicine, 7(1). Retrieved from http://www.medscape.org/viewarticle/497982

Drennen, M. (2012). Vegetable "meat" loaf. Retrieved from http://www.myrecipes.com/recipe/vegetable-meat-loaf-50400000119679

Epel, E., Lapidus, R., McEwen, B., & Brownell, K. (2001). Stress may add bite to appetite in women: A laboratory study of stress induced cortisol and eating behavior. *Psychoneuroendocrinology, 26,* 37-49.

Fry, S. (2012). *Eggs benedict, anyone?* Retrieved fromhttp://www.cookinglight.com/healthy-living/healthy-habits/cooking-light-healthy-habits-program-00412000069559

Gardner, H. (1995). Reflections on multiple intelligences: Myths and messages. *Phi Delta Kappan, 77,* 200-209.

Gardner, H. (1999). *Intelligence reframed: Multiple intelligences for the 21st century.* New York, NY: Basic Books.

Gottfredson, L. S. (2004). Intelligence: Is it the epidemiologists' elusive fundamental cause of social class inequalities in health? *Journal of Personality and Social Psychology, 86*(1), 174-199.

Grow, H. M. G., Cook, A. J., Arterburn, D. E., Saelens, B. E., Drewnowski, A., &

Lozano, P. (2010). Child obesity associated with social disadvantage of children's neighborhoods. *Social Science Medicine, 71*, 584-591.

Gundersen, C., Kreider, B., & Pepper, J. (2012). The impact of the National School Lunch program on child health: A nonparametric bounds analysis. *Journal of Econometrics, 166*, 79-91.

Habif, T. P. *Clinical dermatology: A color guide to diagnosis and therapy* (5th ed.). New York, NY: Mosby Elsevier.

Hatfield, H. (2005). *Emotional eating: Feeding your feelings. Eating to feed a feeling, and not a growling stomach, is emotional eating.* Retrieved from http://www .webmd.com/diet/features/emotional-eating-feeding-your-feelings

Harris, J. L., Schwartz, M. B., & Brownell, K. D. (2010). *Evaluating fast food nutrition and marketing to youth.* New Haven, CT: Rudd Center for Food Policy and Obesity.

Hedley, A. A., Ogden, C. L., Johnson, C. L., Carroll, M. D., Curtin, L. R., & Flegal, K. M. (2010). Prevalence of overweight and obesity among U.S. children, adolescents, and adults, 1999-2002. *JAMA, 291*, 2847-2850. doi:10.1001/jama .291.23.2847

Helm, J. (2011). *Becoming a more mindful eater.* Retrieved from http://www.simmerandboil.cookinglight.com/2011/12/05/becoming-a-more-mindfuk-eater

Henry J. Kaiser Family Foundation. (2004). *The role of media in childhood obesity.* Menlo Park, CA: Author.

Hildegard of Bingen. (2004). *The soul is the greening life force of the flesh.* Retrieved from http://www.friendsofsilence.net/quote/author/hildegard-bingen

Jacobson, M. F. (2012, January/February). Spending to save on obesity. *Nutrition Action Healthletter, 39*(3). Retrieved from http://www.sugarydrinkfacts.org/resources/ sugarydrinkfacts_report.pdf

Lacour, M., & Tissington, L. D. (2011). The effects of poverty on academic achievement. *Educational Research and Reviews,* 6, 522-527.

Ladd, H. F. (2011). Education and poverty: Confronting the evidence (Policy Brief No. 9). Retrieved from http://www.jstor.org/stable/10.1086/649831

Lee, A. G., & Wall, M. (2010). *Idiopathic intracranial hypertension (pseudotumorcerebri): Clinical features and diagnosis.* Retrieved from http://www.update.com/Home/index.html

Mayo Clinic. (2012). *Exchange list: Fruits.* Retrieved from http://www.mayoclinic.com/health/diabetes-diet/DA00070

McLeod, S. A. (2011). *Albert Bandura's social learning theory.* Retrieved from http://www.simplypsychology.org/bandura.html

McLeod, S. A. (2012). Maslow's hierarchy of needs. Retrieved from http://www.simplypsychology.org/maslow.html

Millimet, D. L., Tchernis, R., & Hussain, M. (2008). School nutrition programs and the incidence of childhood obesity. *Journal of Human Resources, 45*, 640-654.

Nguyen-Rodriquez, S. T., Chou, C., Unger, J. B., & Spruijt-Metz, D. (2008). BMI as a moderator of perceived stress and emotional eating in adolescents. *Eating Behavior, 9*, 238-246.

Ogden C. L., Lamb M. M., & Carroll, M. D. (2010). *Obesity and socioeconomic status in children: United States 1988-1994 and 2005-2008* (NCHS Data Brief No. 51). Hyattsville, MD: National Center for Health Statistics.

Ogden, J. (2010). *Health psychology* (2nd ed.). Oxford, United Kingdom: British

Psychological Society and Blackwell.

Piaget, J. *The origin of intelligence in children*. New York, NY: W. W. Norton.

Reeves, D. (2000). *High performance in high poverty schools: 90/90/90 and beyond*. Retrieved from http://www.sabine.k12.la.us/online/leadershipacademy/high%20 performance%20 90%2090%2090%20and%20beyond.pdf

Rhodes, P. (2011, July). Oops! The nutrition edition: 22 common mistakes that can lead anyone astray and how to avoid them for better health. *Cooking Light*, 94-105.

Rodale, Inc. (2008). *Take charge of your health reports.* Retrieved from http://www.au.lifestyle.yahoo.com/prevention/nutrition/galleries/photo/-/14751051/top-6-foods-to-melt-belly-fat/14751052

Salamon, M. (2012, July 16). Poor sleep may age your brain: Inadequate shuteye associated with mental decline in four new studies. *HealthDay News.*

Schanzenbach, D. W. (2005). *Do school lunches contribute to childhood obesity?* Chicago, IL: University of Chicago.

Schardt, D. (2012, April). Sleep on it: When counting sheep isn't enough. *Nutrition Action Healthletter, 39*(3), 9-11.

Sifferlin, A. (2012). *CDC: Higher income and education levels linked to better health.* http://www.healthland.time.com/2012/05/16/cdc-higher-income-and-education-levels-linked-to-better-health/#ixzz24a0yyLBo

Skinner, B. F. (1938). *The behavior of organisms: An experimental analysis.* New York, NY: Appleton-Century-Crofts.

Speiser, P. W., Rudolf, M. C., Anhalt, H., Camacho-Hubner, C., Chiarelli, F., Eliakim, A., . . . Hochberg, Z. (2005). Childhood obesity. *Journal of Clinical Endocrinology and Metabolism, 90*, 1871-1887.

Strasburger, V. C. (2011). Children, adolescents, obesity, and the media (Policy Statement). *Council on Communications and Media Pediatrics, 128*, 201-208.

Strenze, T. (2007). Intelligence and socioeconomic success: A meta-analytic review of longitudinal research. *Intelligence, 35*, 401-426.

United Health Care. (2012). *Annual survey finds more than half of 100-year-olds are exercising nearly every day.* Retrieved from http://www.unitedhealthgroup.com/ newsroom/ news.aspx?id=43dd499e-b7f0-4153-9a87-dbf500bad5d1

U.S. Department of Education. (1992). *The food guide pyramid: A guide to daily food choices.* Retrieved from http://www.nal.usda.gov/fnic/Fpyr.pmap.htm

U.S. Department of Education. (2005). *The food guide pyramid: A guide to daily food choices* (2nd ed.). Retrieved from http://www.nal.usda.gov/fnic/Fpyr.pmap.htm

U.S. Department of Education. (2011). *The food guide pyramid: A guide to daily food choices* (3rd ed.). Retrieved from http://www.nal.usda.gov/fnic/Fpyr.pmap.htm

Vosniadou, S. (2001). *How children learn* (Educational Practice Series 7). Chicago, IL: International Academy of Education and International Bureau of Education.

Vygotsky, L. (1978). *Social development theory.* Retrieved from http://www.learning- theories.com/vygotsky-social-learning-theory.html

Whole Grain Council. (n.d.). *Whole grains from A to Z.* Retrieved from http://www.whole grainscouncil.org/whole-grains-101/whole-grains-a-to-z

Healthy Recipes and More

Sweet Potato Pancakes

Ingredients:

- 1 ½ cups of all-purpose flour
- 3 ½ teaspoons of baking powder
- 1 teaspoon of salt
- ½ teaspoon of ground nutmeg
- ½ teaspoon of cinnamon
- 1 ¼ cups of cooked sweet potatoes - mashed
- 2 eggs - beaten
- 1 ½ cups of milk
- ¼ cup of butter - melted

Preparation:

1. In a large bowl mix flour, baking powder, salt, nutmeg, and cinnamon.
2. In another bowl combine sweet potatoes, eggs, milk, and butter.
3. Combine wet and dry ingredients, and stir until batter is moist.

4. Grease skillet with cooking spray, and turn on to medium heat.
5. Drop batter by tablespoons and fry on the skillet.
6. Flip once so pancake is browned on both sides.
7. Remove from skillet and serve with maple syrup or cinnamon sugar.

Makes about 24 pancakes.

Did you know…?

Sweet potatoes have lots of fiber, especially with the skin on.

Sweet potatoes have nutrients like potassium, iron, and vitamin B-6.

Sweet potatoes are the official vegetable for North Carolina.

Sweet potatoes can be:

- ✓ Baked
- ✓ Steamed
- ✓ Boiled
- ✓ Micro-waved
- ✓ Fried
- ✓ Juiced
- ✓ Pureed
- ✓ Eaten raw

George Washington grew sweet potatoes on his farm in Virginia.

Piggy Buns

Ingredients:

- 1 apple – diced
- 2 eggs - beaten
- 1 cup of milk
- ½ tablespoon of cinnamon
- 8 whole wheat hot dog buns
- 1 cup of cornflakes - crushed
- 8 turkey sausage links

Preparation:

1. Prepare sausage according to package directions and set aside.
2. Crush cornflakes on a plate and set aside.
3. Crack egg in bowl, add milk, and cinnamon. Beat well.
4. Grease skillet with cooking spray, and turn burner on to medium heat.
5. Open each hot dog bun. Dip in egg mixture to cover both sides. Then dip in cornflake crumbs to coat.
6. Place on skillet. Flip once until lightly brown on both sides.
7. Remove from skillet and place on plate to cool. Place sausage in the bun, add diced apples, and maple syrup. Enjoy like a hot dog!

Makes 8 Piggy Buns.

Did you know...?

Don't peel your apple! Most of the fiber and many antioxidants are found in the apple peel.

The largest apple picked weighed three pounds.

Red Delicious, Golden Delicious, Granny Smith, Gala and Fuji are the top five apples eaten in the United States.

Apples are a member of the rose family, along with pears, peaches, plums and cherries.

One apple has five grams of fiber.

Apples are fat, sodium, and cholesterol free.

Antioxidant Muffins

Ingredients:

- 1 ½ cups of all-purpose flour
- ¾ cup of white sugar
- ½ teaspoon of salt
- 2 teaspoons of baking powder
- 1/3 cup of vegetable oil
- 1 egg - beaten
- 1/3 cup of milk
- 1 cup of blueberries
- ½ cup of raspberries
- ½ cup of blackberries

Preparation:

1. Preheat oven to 400 degrees.
2. Line muffin tin with muffin cups.
3. Combine flour, sugar, salt, and baking powder.
4. Place oil into a 1 cup measuring cup. Add the beaten egg and enough milk to fill the cup. Add to flour mixture.
5. Fold in blueberries, raspberries, and blackberries.
6. Fill muffin cups to the top with mix.

7. Bake for 20 to 25 minutes.

Makes about 12 muffins.

Did you know…?

America's favorite muffin is blueberry.

July is national blueberry month.

The blueberry is the official state fruit of New Jersey.

There are over 200 species of raspberries.

Raspberries can be red, black, yellow, or purple.

Blackberries are high in Vitamin C and fiber.

Blackberries are helpful in the treatment of stomach problems.

No-Yolk, Micro-Scrambled Eggs

Ingredients:

- 3 eggs - separated (use only the whites)
- ¼ cup of milk
- ¼ cup of green pepper - diced
- ¼ cup of tomatoes – diced
- ¼ cup of mushrooms - chopped
- ¼ cup of shredded cheddar cheese

Preparation:

1. In a microwaveable bowl, place two egg whites, add milk, and blend with a fork.
2. Add cheese and vegetables to the egg mix.
3. Microwave for 2-3 minutes.
4. Allow eggs to cool for about 1 minute.

Makes 1- 2 servings.

Did you know…?

There are at least 25,000 varieties of tomatoes.

Tomatoes have been called "wolf peach," "a plump thing with a navel," and "the apple of love."

Mushrooms do not need sunshine to grow and thrive.

The pepper is actually a fruit, not a vegetable.

Peppers come in many colors, including green, yellow, orange, red, brown, and purple.

Super Sweet Fruit Salad

Ingredients:

- 1 cup strawberries - diced
- 1 cup blueberries
- 1 cup red grapes - diced
- 1 nectarine - diced
- 1 pear - diced
- 1 apple – diced
- ½ cup of honey
- 1 ½ cups of fruit juice (grape, apple, orange, cranberry, or any other kind - you choose!)
- ½ lemon or ½ an orange
- *Optional:* nuts, raisins, or other dried fruit

Preparation:

1. Wash fruit. Chop or dice each fruit into bite-sized pieces and place in a large bowl.
2. Pour juice on top and add honey.

3. Squeeze the juice of ½ of one lemon or ½ of one orange on top of the fruit.
4. Stir gently until fruit and juices are mixed well.

Makes about 8-10 servings.

Did you know...?

Nectarines don't have fuzz but peaches do.

Nectarines are an excellent source of vitamins A and C.

In China, it's bad luck to share a pear.

Pear's nickname is "butter fruit."

Grapes can come in many colors, like white, red, black, blue, green, purple and golden.

Grapes are on the top ten list of favorite fruits.

Over 80% of strawberries are grown in California.

Strawberries are hand-picked because they are so fragile.

Cowboy Banana Smoothies

Ingredients:

- 2 bananas
- 6-8 strawberries
- 1 cup of peach yogurt
- 1 ½ cups of mango juice or mango nectar

Preparation:

1. Fill blender pitcher 1/3 of the way with ice cubes.
2. Pour mango juice over ice.
3. Add yogurt, bananas, and strawberries.
4. Cover and blend until liquefied.

Makes about 6 servings.

Did you know…?

Bananas, apples, and watermelons float in water.

The average American eats 27 pounds of bananas each year!

An individual banana is called a finger. A bunch of bananas is called a hand.

Bananas are a good source of vitamin B6, which your brain needs to function properly and make you wise.

Mangoes are related to cashews and pistachios

The mango is a symbol of love in India.

Melon Kabobs and Yogurt Dip

Ingredients:

- ½ of a honeydew melon
- ½ of a small watermelon
- ½ of a cantaloupe
- ½ of a mush melon
- 1 ½ cups vanilla yogurt
- ½ cup honey
- Juice of ½ lime

Preparation:

1. Slice off rind of each melon and cut into large bite-sized chunks.
2. Place melon in various patterns on wooden skewers.
3. In a small bowl, mix yogurt, honey, and lime.
4. Use skewers to dip melon chunks in yogurt dip.
5. Try other fruits too!

Makes 6-8 servings.

Did you know...?

Honeydew melons are also known as temptation melons.

Honeydews are the sweetest of all melons when ripe.

Cantaloupe is a great source of Vitamin A.

Most cantaloupes are grown in Arizona or California.

Watermelon is 92% water.

Watermelon is usually red, but there is also a yellow variety.

Sweet & Crunchy Veggie Salad

Ingredients:

- 4 cups of lettuce - shredded
- 1 cup of raw green beans - diced
- 1 cup of raw carrots - diced
- ½ cup of raw jicama - diced
- ½ cup of raw white onion - diced
- ½ cup of blue cheese chunks
- ½ cup of dried cranberries
- ¼ cup of pecans – chopped

Dressing:

- ¼ cup of maple syrup
- ½ cup of white vinegar
- 1 tablespoon of sugar
- Juice of ½ lemon

Preparation:

1. Slice the vegetables, place them in a large bowl, and set aside.
2. In a separate bowl, make dressing: Mix vinegar, maple syrup, sugar, and lemon. Blend well.
3. Add cheese, dried fruit, and nuts.
4. Pour dressing over salad mix and toss until well coated.

Makes about 4-6 servings.

Did you know…?

Lettuce is a member of the sunflower family.

Dark green lettuce leaves are more nutritious than lighter green leaves.

Green beans are a great source of fiber.

The heaviest carrot on record was nearly 19 pounds.

The longest carrot on record was 16 feet 10.5 inches long.

Jicama is a member of the potato family and can weigh up to 50 pounds.

Onions can heal blisters.

Fun Fiesta Salsa

Ingredients:

- 4 medium sized tomatoes - diced
- ½ green pepper - diced
- ½ red pepper - diced
- ½ yellow pepper - diced
- 1 white onion - diced
- ½ cup of vinegar

- 1 tablespoon of cilantro
- 1 teaspoon of garlic salt
- 1 teaspoon of black pepper
- Juice of ½ lemon or ½ lime
- Tortilla chips – like blue corn chips, or quinoa chips

Preparation:

1. Dice vegetables and place in a large bowl.
2. Pour vinegar over vegetables.
3. Add cilantro, garlic salt, black pepper, and lemon or lime juice.
4. Mix well, chill, and serve with tortilla chips.

Makes about 10-12 servings.

Did you know...?

Peppers are actually fruits that form on the plant after it flowers.
Peppers can be green, red, yellow, and orange.
Sometimes peppers can even be white, purple, blue, and brown, depending on when they are harvested.
Tomatoes are actually a fruit.
Tomato season is from June to November.
Onion can help remove warts.
Onions can soothe an insect bite.

Hayden's Tasty Guac

Ingredients:

- 2 avocados - sliced
- 2 tomatoes – diced
- 1 yellow onion - diced
- 1 can sweet corn - drained

- 1 can black beans - drained
- Juice of ½ lemon
- Garlic salt
- Black pepper
- ¼ cup white vinegar

Preparation:

1. In a large bowl, mash avocados with a fork.
2. Add tomatoes, onions, sweet corn, and beans.
3. Add juice of ½ lemon, garlic salt, black pepper, and vinegar.
4. Mix well, chill, and serve with tortilla chips.

Makes about 8-10 servings.

Did you know…?

San Diego is the avocado capital of the U.S.

Varieties of avocados include Bacon, Fuerte, Gwen, Hass, Macarthur, Pinkerton, Reed, and Zulano.

Corn is available in yellow, white, red, and blue.

Corn is also known as maize.

Onions can help cure the common cold.

Egyptians worshipped onions. They believed the onion symbolized eternal life.

Roasted Veggie Salad

Ingredients:

- 1 zucchini - cubed
- 6 asparagus stalks - sliced
- 1 cup of baby carrots

- 2 red bell peppers - diced
- 1 sweet potato - cubed
- 3 potatoes - cubed
- ¼ cup of olive oil
- 2 tablespoons of balsamic vinegar
- garlic salt, salt, and black pepper

Preparation:

1. Preheat oven to 475 degrees.
2. In a large bowl, combine all vegetables.
3. In a small bowl, stir together olive oil, vinegar, salt, and pepper.
4. Toss oil mix with vegetables until they are all coated.
5. Spread evenly on a large roasting pan.
6. Sprinkle garlic salt, salt, and black pepper over the vegetables.
7. Roast for 35 to 40 minutes in the oven, stirring every 10 minutes or until vegetables are cooked through and browned.

Makes about 6-8 servings.

Did you know…?

A zucchini has more potassium than a banana.

The word zucchini comes from "zucca" the Italian word for squash.

The name, asparagus, comes from the Greek language and means "sprout" or "shoot."

Asparagus is a member of the Lily family.

In 1974, a man grew 370 pounds of potatoes on one plant.

Buds on potatoes are called "eyes."

The world's largest potato chip measured 23 feet x 14.5 feet.

Go Green! Raw Slaw

Ingredients:

- 2 cups of broccoli - chopped
- 1 cup of green beans - chopped
- 1 cup snow peas - chopped
- 1 cup cabbage – chopped
- 1 green pepper - chopped
- 2 cups of fat free sour cream
- ½ cup of white sugar
- ¼ cup of vinegar

Preparation:

1. Chop raw vegetables into small pieces and place in a bowl.
2. Add sour cream, sugar, and vinegar.
3. Mix well and serve cold.

Makes 4-6 servings.

Did you know…?

The average person in the United States eats four and one half pounds of broccoli each year.

Broccoli got its name from the Latin word *bracchium*, which means strong arm or branch. They look like little trees!

California and Arizona produced 100% of the national total.

Cabbage can be purple or green.

Cabbage can improve digestion.

The snow pea is also called the "China mangetout."

Lettuce Eat! Tuna Salad Sandwiches

Ingredients:

- 2 cans chunk light tuna in water
- 1 white onion, diced
- 2 cups of fat free sour cream
- ½ cup of alfalfa sprouts or bean sprouts
- 6-10 leaves of lettuce
- Whole wheat crackers
- Salt and pepper to taste

Preparation:

1. Open tuna cans carefully and drain off water.
2. Place tuna in bowl. Add onion, sour cream, salt and pepper to taste. Mix well.
3. Rinse lettuce leaves and dry thoroughly.
4. Place one piece of lettuce on a plate.
5. Scoop a large serving of the tuna salad onto the lettuce leaf, and top with alfalfa sprouts or bean sprouts.
6. Roll up lettuce leaf to make a tuna wrap. Or, use wheat crackers to make mini tuna sandwiches.

Makes about 6-8 servings.

Did you know...?

Alfalfa is really a member of the pea family.
Alfalfa sprouts is the top source of anti-oxidant among all vegetables.
Alfalfa sprouts have nutrients like calcium, folic acid, magnesium, manganese, potassium, silicon, sodium, and zinc.
Tuna fish can flush toxins out of your liver.
Tuna fish is high in Vitamins A, B, and E.
Tuna fish is low in fat and is a fat-burning powerhouse.

Ba-gawk! Chicken Salad Sandwich/Wrap

Ingredients:

- 2 cups of chicken – cooked and diced
- ¾ cup mayonnaise
- 1 teaspoon of mustard
- 2 eggs – hardboiled and chopped
- ½ cup of celery - diced
- ¼ cup of red onion - diced
- ½ cup of green grapes - chopped
- 4-6 whole wheat tortilla wraps

Preparation:

1. Cook chicken according to package directions (or used canned or pre-cooked chicken). Chop into bite-sized pieces.
2. In a large bowl, mix chicken, mayonnaise, mustard, salt and pepper to taste.
3. Add hardboiled eggs, diced vegetables and chopped grapes.
4. Mix gently and thoroughly.
5. Spoon some chicken salad onto a tortilla wrap and roll it up.

Makes 4-6 servings.

Did you know…?

Chicken is low in fat and high in protein, so it's a good source of energy.

Chicken contains Vitamins B and E., and other nutrients like riboflavin, niacin, and thiamin.

A bunch of celery is called a "stalk." Each piece is called a "rib."

Medieval magicians put celery seeds in their shoes in order to fly.
Grapes can be green, red, and blue including: Fantasy, Flame, Red Globe, Ribier and Thompson.

Bacon Lover's Sandwich

Ingredients:

- 2 slices of whole wheat bread
- 2 slices of lean turkey lunchmeat
- 2 slices of low sodium bacon
- 2 slices of avocado
- 2 slices of tomato
- 2 slices of cheese – provolone or cheddar (or both!)

Preparation:

1. Cook bacon according to package directions and set aside to cool.
2. Slice avocado and tomato.
3. Toast 2 slices of bread.
4. Top toasted bread with cheese slices.
5. Add bacon, tomato, avocado, and turkey.

Makes 1 whole sandwich.

Did you know...?

Bacon is a good source of protein, niacin, phosphorus and selenium.
September 3rd is international bacon day.
Turkey breast lunch meat is a good source of protein.
Whole wheat bread has roughly 3 times the fiber of white bread.
Cheese contains calcium and other vitamins and minerals which are good for your bones and teeth.

Gimme 5! Bean Salad

Ingredients:

- 1 15 oz. can of garbanzo beans
- 1 15 oz. can pinto beans
- 1 15 oz. can black beans
- 1 15 oz. can kidney beans
- 1 15 oz. can cannellini beans
- 1 cup of white vinegar
- 1 cup of sugar
- 3/4 cup of olive oil

Preparation:

1. Open cans carefully.
2. Rinse beans with cold water and place them in a large bowl.
3. In a separate bowl, mix vinegar, sugar, and oil to make dressing.
4. Pour dressing over the top of the beans.
5. Mix well, chill and serve cold.

Makes 10-12 servings.

Did you know…?

Beans could be called, "healthy people's meat."

Beans can help reduce heart attacks.

The pinto bean has more protein than any other bean.

Pinto beans are also called, "frijoles."

Black beans are also known as turtle beans, French beans, black kidney beans, black Mexican beans, and Mexican beans

Cannellini beans are also called, "white kidney beans."

Baked Potato Salad

Ingredients:

- 4 baking potatoes
- 2 cups of fat free sour cream
- 2 cups of shredded cheddar cheese
- 5 slices of bacon - crumbled
- 4 green onions - chopped
- 2 cups of broccoli - chopped

Preparation:

1. Wash vegetables.
2. Poke potatoes with a fork several times.
3. Cook potatoes in microwave for 5 minutes. Use an oven mitt to flip over hot potatoes. Microwave for 5 more minutes.
4. Allow potatoes to cool, carefully cut into bite-sized pieces, and place in a large bowl.
5. Add shredded cheese, sour cream, green onions, broccoli, and bacon crumbles.
6. Mix well. Serve warm or cold.

Makes about 8 servings.

Did you know…?

In 1995, the potato was the first vegetable to be grown in space.

You can put slices of raw potato on broken bones to speed healing.

French fries were introduced in the states when Thomas Jefferson was in office between the years of 1801-1809.

Eating potatoes with other foods can prevent indigestion.

Potato chips were invented in 1853.

Gyro Pasta Salad

Ingredients:

- 1 box of spiral pasta
- 1 pound of lean ground beef
- 1 cucumber - diced
- 1 tomato - diced
- ½ white onion - diced
- 2 cups of sour cream
- 1 teaspoon of garlic salt
- Salt and pepper to taste
- 1 head of lettuce, ripped into small pieces
- Pita bread, sliced into strips

Preparation:

1. Cook pasta according to directions.
2. Drain noodles and place in a large bowl.
3. Add sour cream, garlic salt, and pepper. Mix well.
4. Cook lean ground beef and drain off grease. Add to noodles.
5. Add cucumber, tomato, and onion.
6. Mix well.
7. Serve on a bed of lettuce with a side of pita bread strips.

Makes about 8 servings.

Did you know…?

Beef contains protein that can help build muscle.

Beef has zinc, Vitamin B12, and iron.

Lean beef has more Vitamin B12, more zinc, and more iron than the same size serving of skinless chicken breast.

The flavor of a cucumber comes from its seeds.

The inside of a cucumber can be up to 20 degrees cooler than the outside air.

Ricardo's Mexican Pasta Salad

Ingredients:

- 1 box of wheel pasta
- 2 cups of shredded cheddar cheese
- 2 cups of fat free sour cream
- 1 taco seasoning packet
- 1 tomato - diced
- 1 green pepper - diced
- 5 green onions - diced
- 3 cups of cooked chicken - diced
- ½ can of black olives
- 1 can of black beans - rinsed
- Taco chips

Preparation:

1. Cook pasta according to directions, drain with water, and place in a large bowl.
2. Add cheese, sour cream, and taco seasoning packet. Mix well.
3. Add tomato, green pepper, onion, chicken, olives, and beans. Mix well again, stirring gently.
4. Serve on a bed of taco chips.

Makes about 8 servings.

Did you know...?

Chinese people were making noodles as early as 3000 BC.

Noodles are low in fat and low in sodium.

The average American eats 20 pounds of pasta each year.

Tomatoes can lower your risk of cancer.

In the U.S., tomatoes are eaten more than any other fruit or vegetable.

Florida is the number one producer of fresh market tomatoes.

Lean Burger Pasta Salad

Ingredients:

- 1 box of macaroni pasta
- 1 ½ cups of mayonnaise
- 2 cups of shredded cheddar cheese
- 1 pound of lean ground beef
- 1 cup of dill pickle chips
- 1 tomato - diced
- 1 onion - diced
- 1 head of lettuce - shredded
- Ketchup
- Mustard
- Potato sticks or potato chips

Preparation:

1. Cook pasta according to directions, drain, and place in a large bowl.
2. Add mayo and cheese. Mix well.
3. Cook lean ground beef, drain off grease, and add to noodles.
4. Add tomato, onion, and dill pickle chips. Mix well.
5. Serve on a bed of lettuce, and top with potato sticks.
6. Add a decorative squirt of ketchup and mustard on top.

Makes 6-8 servings.

Did you know…?

In America, dill pickles are twice as popular as sweet pickles.

The largest hamburger on record weighed 5,000 pounds.

The average American eats 3 hamburgers per week.

The first fast-food burger made in 1921 cost 5 cents.

The Hamburger Hall of Fame is located in Wisconsin.

Mystery of the Missing Tomato Pesto

Ingredients:

- 1 box of angel hair pasta
- 2 large tomatoes - chopped
- 1 cup of olive oil
- 1 tablespoon of garlic salt
- ½ cup of parmesan cheese
- 3 cups of green beans - raw or cooked

Preparation:

1. Cook pasta according to directions, drain, and set aside.
2. In a blender, mix tomatoes, olive oil, garlic salt, and parmesan cheese until well blended.
3. Pour tomato pesto over angel hair pasta.
4. Serve warm or cold with a side of fresh green beans.

Makes 4-6 servings.

Did you know…?

The Aztecs made what may be the first salsa - tomatoes prepared with peppers, corn, and salt.

China is the world's largest producer of tomatoes.

The leaves of a tomato plant are poisonous.

Green beans can actually be green, yellow, purple, or speckled in those colors.

Green beans vary in size, but the average length is about 4 inches.

Gino's Homemade Pizza

Ingredients:

- 1 package of yeast
- 2 ½ cups of flour
- ½ teaspoon of garlic salt
- 2 tablespoons of oil
- 2-3 cups of shredded mozzarella cheese
- 2 cups of tomato sauce
- ½ cup of mushrooms - sliced
- ½ cup of green peppers - diced
- ½ cup of pineapples - diced
- Pepperoni slices

Preparation:

1. Dissolve yeast in 1 cup of warm water (not too hot, not too cold).
2. Add flour, garlic salt, and oil. Knead until dough forms.
3. Cover and let dough rise for 10 minutes.
4. Roll out dough with rolling pin. Place in pie pan. Poke holes in dough with a fork. Pre-cook dough in 375 degree oven for about 7 minutes.
5. Carefully remove dough from oven. Add sauce, cheese, and toppings of your choice. Return to oven and cook for 12 minutes.
6. Remove cooked pizza from oven and allow it to cool before serving.

Makes two large pizzas.

Did you know...?

Throughout history, mushrooms were thought to have medicinal powers.

Peppers are a good source of Vitamin C.

There are four types of pineapples including Gold, smooth Cayenne, Red Spanish and Sugar Loaf.

A pineapple can weigh up to 10 pounds.

A pineapple takes about 18 months to grow.

Nana's Left-over Turkey and Vegetable Soup

Ingredients:

- 2 cups of roasted turkey - chopped into bite sized chunks
- 2 cups of turkey broth
- 2 cups of carrots - diced
- 1 yellow onion - diced
- 4 celery stalks - diced
- 1 can of corn - rinsed
- 2 cups of cabbage - diced
- 1 cup of lima beans
- 1 tablespoon of garlic salt
- Pepper
- Salt

Preparation:

1. Dice vegetables and place them together in a large bowl.
2. In a large cooking pot, pour 2 cups of turkey broth, 4 cups of water, and garlic salt. Bring to a boil.
3. Carefully add vegetables and turkey chunks.

4. Turn down to low heat and let the soup simmer for 20 minutes.
5. Add salt and pepper to taste.
6. Serve with whole wheat crackers or oyster crackers.

Makes 8-10 servings.

Did you know…?

Lima beans are rich source of antioxidants, vitamins, minerals, and fiber.

Carrots help improve eyesight, especially at night.

Carrots help keep your skin and hair healthy.

Carrots have the highest beta-carotene of any vegetable.

Holtville, California dubs itself "The Carrot Capital of the World."

The largest cabbage on record weighed 123 pounds.

A cabbage can grow in three months time.

Crumb's Cornflake Chicken and Sweet Potato Bakes

Ingredients:

- 1 ½ cups of cornflakes - crushed
- 8-10 chicken tenderloins
- 1 egg
- ½ cup of milk
- ¾ cup of parmesan cheese
- 2 large sweet potatoes
- 1 cup butter
- Brown sugar
- Cinnamon

Preparation:

1. In a small bowl, mix egg and milk until well blended. In another bowl, crush cornflakes and mix with parmesan cheese.
2. Grease a small baking dish. Use a fork to dip the chicken in the egg mix, then the cornflake mix, and place in the baking dish.
3. Place chicken in oven at 350 degrees and cook for 20 minutes.
4. Chop sweet potatoes into bite-sized wedges. Mix with butter, sugar, and cinnamon. Microwave for 5 minutes.
5. Remove from microwave and pour into a greased baking dish. Cook in a 350 degree oven for 10 minutes.

Makes 8-10 servings.

Did you know…?

Milk contains proteins, calcium, phosphorus, magnesium, and potassium.

Milk promotes healthy skin and eyes.

The sweet potato is a part of the morning glory family.

Sweet potatoes are also called "yams."

There are three types of sweet potatoes grown: rose or red-skinned, orange-fleshed, and white or tan-fleshed.

Cheesy Mac and Veggies

Ingredients:

- 1 (16 oz.) package of macaroni
- 2 cups of shredded cheddar cheese
- 1 cup of Havarti cheese
- 2 tablespoons of parmesan cheese
- 2 ½ cup of milk
- 3 tablespoons of margarine
- 2 cups of chicken broth
- 1 small tomato – diced
- 1 cup of broccoli – diced
- 2 cups of green beans

Preparation:

1. Cook the macaroni according to the package directions, rinse, and place in a lightly-greased, oven-safe bowl. Mix in broccoli and tomato.
2. In a saucepan over low heat, melt the margarine. Add the chicken broth and milk.
3. Stir in the cheese, saving a little to sprinkle on top. Stir until cheese is melted then pour over macaroni.
4. Bake for 30 minutes at 350 degrees.
5. Serve with a side of green beans.

Makes 4-6 servings.

Did you know…?

There is a crayon color called "macaroni and cheese."

There are two restaurants in New York that serve only macaroni and cheese.

Macaroni and cheese is the number one cheese recipe in the United States.
Macaroni and cheese is one of the top ten comfort foods in the United States.
Kraft sells more than one million boxes of macaroni and cheese every day.

Ghetti and Turkey Meatballs

Ingredients:

- 1 pound of ground turkey
- 1 egg
- ½ cup of potato chips - crushed
- Garlic salt, salt, and black pepper to taste
- 1 16.oz package of spaghetti
- I jar of pasta sauce
- 1 large tomato – diced
- ½ white onion - diced

Preparation:

1. In a glass bowl, mix the ground turkey egg, bread crumbs and a sprinkle of garlic salt, pepper, and salt.
2. With your hands, shape the meat into balls. Cook in a skillet at medium heat until fully cooked (about 5-8 minutes). Drain fat.
3. Cook spaghetti according to package directions. Drain.
4. Warm pasta sauce, Add onions and tomatoes.
5. Place spaghetti on plate, top with sauce and meatballs.

Makes about 6 servings.

Did you know…?

There are 42 calories in one turkey meatball.

Meatballs can be made with beef, chicken, turkey, or pork.

Many nations and cultures make meatballs with their own kinds of sauces and gravies.

Originally, meatballs were served alone and spaghetti was served alone. It wasn't until much later that the two were served together.

In Afghanistan, meatballs are not grilled and placed on top of pizza.

In October 2009 an Italian eatery in Concord, New Hampshire set the record for the biggest meatball at 222.5 pounds.

Chinese rice with tofu/Vegetable stir fry

Ingredients:

- 1 package whole grain rice
- 1 cup tofu – firm, chopped
- 1 cup cabbage – shredded or chopped
- 1 cup bok choy - chopped
- 1 cup green onion - diced
- 1 cup carrots - diced
- 1 cup green peppers - diced
- 1 cup broccoli - chopped
- ¼ cup of soy sauce
- ½ cup of olive oil

Preparation:

1. Cook rice according to package directions. Set aside.

2. In a large skillet or wok, warm olive oil to medium heat.
3. Add tofu and cook until lightly browned.
4. Add vegetables, garlic salt, and soy sauce then stir.
5. Cover and steam in pan for 3 minutes.
6. Serve vegetables over rice. Season with soy sauce.

Makes about 8 servings.

Did you know…?

Bok choy is also known as Chinese cabbage.

Bok choy is very nutritious, it's high in Vitamin A, Vitamin C, potassium and calcium.

Tofu acts like a sponge and has the miraculous ability to soak up any flavor that is added to it.

Tofu is also known as soybean curd.

Green onions are also known as scallions.

On a green onion, the white bulb and the green stalk are both edible.

Nana's Apple Pecan Pie

Ingredients:

- 2 tablespoons of flour
- 1 cup of sugar
- ¼ cup of pecans – chopped
- ½ teaspoon of cinnamon
- 6 Red Delicious apples – peeled and sliced
- 1 ½ tablespoons of butter
- 2 ready-made pie crusts

Preparation:

1. In a large bowl, combine flour, sugar, pecans, and cinnamon.
2. Add apple slices and mix well.
3. Place one pie crust dough piece in a 9 inch pie pan.
4. Pour in apple mixture.
5. Cover with second pie dough.
6. Melt butter and brush on top of the pie crust.
7. Bake at 350 degrees for 45 minutes.

Makes about 8 servings.

Did you know…?

The science of apple growing is called pomology.

An American eats about 19 pounds of apples every year.

It takes the energy from 50 leaves to produce one apple.

The largest apple ever picked weighed three pounds, two ounces.

The skin of an apple contains more antioxidants and fiber than the flesh.

The apple is the official state fruit of Washington, New York, Rhode Island, and West Virginia.

China produces more apples than any other country.

Healthy Benji's Mix Mania

Ingredients:

- ½ cup of raisins
- ½ cup of chocolate chips
- 1 cup of cereal pieces – like Cheerios, Rice Chex, or Kix
- ½ cup of dried cranberries
- ½ cup of dried blueberries

- ½ cup of dried fruit pieces – like apricots, bananas, or mangos
- ½ cup of peanuts or almond
- 1 cup of pretzel sticks
- ½ cup of mini marshmallows
- ½ cup of goldfish crackers

Preparation:

1. Open a ½ gallon zip-close bag.
2. Add raisins, chocolate chips, cranberries, blueberries, dried fruit, and nuts.
3. Close bag and shake to mix.
4. Open bag and add the cereal pieces, pretzels, marshmallows, and crackers.
5. Close bag and shake to mix again.

Makes about 10 servings.

Did you know…?

Cranberries are a good source of Vitamin C.

Another name for cranberries is "bounceberries" because they bounce when they are ripe.

Cranberries are grown on sandy bogs or marshes. Because cranberries float, some bogs are flooded when the fruit is ready for harvesting.

Michigan is the nation's top producer of blueberries.

Apricots are a good source of Vitamins A and C, as well as potassium and fiber.

Tutti Fruity Ice Cream Pie

Ingredients:

- 3 cups vanilla frozen yogurt
- ½ cup of fresh or frozen cherries – pitted
- ½ cup of fresh peaches – diced
- ½ cup of pineapple - diced
- 1 chocolate-cookie pie crust

Preparation:

1. In a large bowl, combine ice cream, cherries, peaches, and pineapples. Stir gently to mix.
2. Pour mix into the graham cracker crust.
3. Freeze until the pie is firm, at least 4 hours.

Makes about 8 servings.

Did you know...?

There are two kinds of cherries – tart and sweet.

Tart cherries can help relieve a headache.

Michigan produces the most cherries of any state.

The pineapple was first called, "anana" which is the Caribbean word for "excellent fruit."

The pineapple is actually a cluster of 100-200 fruitlets.

The world's largest peach weighed 10,000 pounds.

Georgia is known as the Peach State.

Make the breakfast drink that Dr. Oz swears by! This "green drink" is high in fiber, low-calorie and rich in vitamins.

Ingredients

- 2 cups spinach
- 1/2 cucumber
- 1/4 head of celery
- 1/2 bunch parsley
- 1 bunch mint
- 3 carrots
- 2 apples
- 1/4 orange
- 1/4 lime
- 1/4 lemon
- 1/4 pineapple

Directions

Combine all ingredients in a blender. This makes approximately 28-30 ounces, or 3-4 servings.

APPENDIX

Additional Related Websites

http://www.myrecipes.com/recipe/potato-root-vegetable-mashers-50400000119694

http://www.myrecipes.com/recipe/cajun-stufed-potatoes-50400000119696

http://www.nationaldairycouncil.org/Pages/Home.aspx

http://www.nourishinteracive.com/healthy-living/family-nutrition-exercise-facts/healthy-food-choices-family/protein-food-group/protein-products

http://www.wholegrainscouncil.org/whole-grains-101/whole-grains-a-to-z

http://www.wholegrainnation.eatbetteramerica.com

http://www.choosemyplate.gov/healthy-eating-tips/ten-tips.html

http://www.choosemyplate.gov/food-groups/dairy-counts.html

http://www.doctoroz.com/recipes

The Must Knows

Blood Pressure

In adults (measured in millimeters of mercury, or mmHg)

Category	Systolic (top number)		Diastolic (bottom number)
Normal	Less than 120	&	Less than 80
Prehypertension	120-139	or	80-89

High Blood Pressure

Stage 1	140-159	or	90-99
Stage 2	160 or higher	or	100 or higher

Cholesterol Levels

Total cholesterol level

• Less than 200 mg/dL	Desirable
• 200-239 mg/dL	Borderline High
• 240 mg/dL or higher	High

Total cholesterol is the level of all of the lipids in your blood, including your LDL-cholesterol and HDL-cholesterol. Generally, a lower total cholesterol level is better.

LDL-Cholesterol

• Less than 100 mg/dL	Optimal
• 100-129 mg/dL	Near Optimal
• 130-159 mg/dL	Borderline High
• 160-189 mg/dL	High
• 190 mg/dL or higher	Very High

LDL-cholesterol is considered the "bad" cholesterol because if you have too much LDL-cholesterol in your bloodstream, it can lead to plaque buildup in your arteries over time, known as atherosclerosis. Generally a lower LDL-cholesterol level is better.

HDL-Cholesterol

• 60 mg/dL or higher	High
• Less than 40 mg/dL	Low

HDL-cholesterol is considered the "good" cholesterol because it helps return cholesterol to the liver, where it can be eliminated from the body. Generally, a higher HDL-cholesterol level is better.

Triglycerides

• Less than 150 mg/dL	Normal
• 150-199 mg/dL	Borderline high
• 200-499 mg/dL	High
• 500 mg/dL or higher	Very high

Triglycerides, like cholesterol, are another substance that can be dangerous to your health. Like LDL-cholesterol, you want to keep your triglycerides low.

Source: National Cholesterol Education Program (NCEP)

Body Mass Index...page 43

Index

About the Author

Dr. Verna R. Benjamin-Lambert has dedicated her life to serving children. Her tireless passion to help the youth is fueled by her strong belief that given a chance, every child can experience success.

A graduate of St. Joseph's Teachers' College in her native country of Jamaica, West Indies, she migrated to the United States where she worked in the private sector before returning to the classroom. Her studies at Kennesaw State University in psychology, and West Georgia University in Special Education Leadership, gave her the tools to become an advocate for students with disabilities. Following her undergraduate studies, she went on to obtain her doctorate from Nova Southeastern University.

As an administrator at one of the leading school systems in Georgia, she became a voice for children who were being left behind in the academic setting. She retired from the school system to fulfill a lifetime goal of establishing The Benjamin Preschool of Academic and Performing Arts in Smyrna, Georgia. Her passion to support children facing challenges led her to author the book, Health Intelligence, a work that grapples with the core issues leading to the obesity crisis among children. Her interest in children's health led to her development of the Healthy Benji series of children's books focused on establishing healthy eating habits in children.

Dr. Benjamin-Lambert is the mother of four successful girls and grandmother of four boys. She enjoys life with her best friend and loving husband, Harry Lambert, Jr., in Kennesaw, Georgia. She is proud to be a citizen of the United States but returns to Jamaica quite frequently to visit her mother and father, Pearly Mae and Albert Benjamin, who she thanks for serving as strong role models for her and her eight siblings.

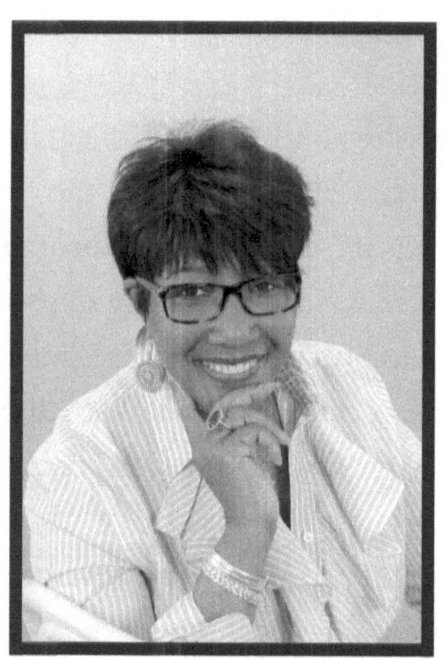

www.ingramcontent.com/pod-product-compliance
Lightning Source LLC
Chambersburg PA
CBHW030300290526
45785CB00001B/159

* 9 7 8 1 4 5 2 5 7 5 6 4 3 *